# Healing the Fragmented U.S. Healthcare System

Through a systems perspective, this insightful book challenges the current state of healthcare in the United States, arguing for overarching reforms that would lead ultimately to universal healthcare coverage across the country.

Written by the president of the board of trustees of a rural hospital, the book highlights the chronic issues facing American healthcare today, namely high costs, poor health outcomes, excessive health inequalities, and a lack of trust. It uses systems thinking principles – used in hospitals themselves to improve efficiency, quality, and safety of care – to show how the fragmented system could be transformed by addressing these issues holistically. The book also gives suggestions for rebuilding trust, respect, and mutual cooperation, issues which are also critical in healing the current system.

Grounded in the author's direct experience in facing the challenges of dealing with a fragmented system in America today, this perceptive book will interest graduate students in healthcare administration, policy, or leadership programs, as well as scholars in these and related fields.

**Barbara J. Sowada** is president of the board of trustees of a rural hospital. She has a Ph.D. in nutrition from Colorado State University. She lives in southwest Wyoming. This is her second book about healthcare reform.

# Healing the Fragmented U.S. Healthcare System

## Bold Solutions for Systemic Problems

**Barbara J. Sowada**

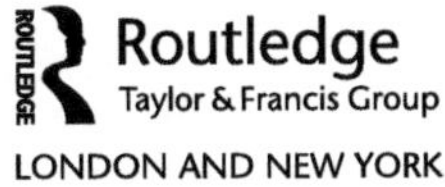


LONDON AND NEW YORK

First published 2025
by Routledge
4 Park Square, Milton Park, Abingdon, Oxon OX14 4RN

and by Routledge
605 Third Avenue, New York, NY 10158

*Routledge is an imprint of the Taylor & Francis Group, an informa business*



*British Library Cataloguing-in-Publication Data*
A catalogue record for this book is available from the British Library

ISBN: 978-1-032-88520-9 (hbk)
ISBN: 978-1-032-96700-4 (pbk)
ISBN: 978-1-003-53822-6 (ebk)

DOI: 10.4324/9781003538226

Typeset in Times New Roman
by KnowledgeWorks Global Ltd.

**For those who work to make healthcare better for everyone.**

# Contents

# Figures

# Introduction

## The System Is the Problem

From cradle to grave, healthcare plays a vital role in our lives. We depend on healthcare for healthy babies and children, care when we are sick or injured, management of our chronic diseases, and comfort at the end of our lives. Good health is a precious personal asset; it definitely makes life less burdensome. Healthy people are vibrant, engaged, productive, and able to participate fully in family activities and in their communities. It's in society's best interest to help everyone stay healthy, for healthy people are critical to a strong economy, social stability, and national security.

Part of being healthy is having access to good healthcare. But, what if our healthcare system isn't so good? The four hallmarks of a high functioning system are (1) it's efficient, it doesn't waste resources; (2) it's effective, its product is good; (3) it's equitable, it's fair, and (4) it fulfills its purpose, healthy people. The U.S. healthcare system violates all four hallmarks. The U.S. healthcare system is inefficient; it is the most expensive in the world. The average per capita spending for Americans is twice that of peer countries, $12,555 compared with the peer countries' average of $6,651.[1] As a $4.5 trillion dollar enterprise, it's better at producing wealth than health. It's ineffective; by almost every metric, the health status of Americans is poorer than that of citizens of similar wealthy countries. And, the system is unfair. Roughly thirty million adults and nine million children don't have health insurance. Plus, there are indisputable health disparities associated with systemic race and income inequities. Finally, its purpose—to improve the health of individuals and communities—has come under question due to the growing role of financial markets, motives, and investors within the healthcare sector.

What if, as W. Edward Deming states, the design of our healthcare system is the problem? This book looks at healthcare's problems through the lens of systems thinking. As we will see in the following chapters, the things we don't like about healthcare—its high costs; its poor health outcomes; its inequitable access to care and distribution of resources—are baked into the structure of the U.S. healthcare system. This book assumes W. Edwards Deming is correct; the problem is the *system*. To solve healthcare's problems is to *redesign* the structure of the U.S. healthcare system.

DOI: 10.4324/9781003538226-1

## Redesigning the System Is the Solution

Redesign means a radical change to the structure of the U.S. healthcare system. Redesign does not mean remodel. Remodel is like updating a kitchen in an older house or replacing a leaking roof but maintaining the original structure of the house. Redesign does not mean piecemeal improvements or incremental reform, for they are the same as remodel. In fact, remodeling healthcare system has made things worse. Since 1970, there've been multiple, intermittent efforts to control healthcare costs, ranging from managed care, competition, consolidation, value-based purchasing, to prior authorization, to name a few. The result, fifty years of continuous cost increases. Between 1970 and 2020, healthcare costs rose from $74.1 billion to $4.1 trillion, respectively.[2] Despite the huge increase in spending, health outcomes have not improved, and for some groups of Americans, health outcomes have gotten worse.

*Bold Solutions for Systemic Problems: Healing a Fractured Healthcare System* looks at the problems of the U.S. healthcare system—it's inefficiencies, ineffectiveness, and inequities—through the lens of systems thinking. Ironically, hospitals are adept at using systems thinking principles to make processes more efficient and improve the quality and safety of care. However, these principles haven't been used for systemic reform.

This book is based on two premises. One is for any system to be improved, there must be agreement on its purpose and assurance the structure of system is composed of the right parts, in the right arrangement, and connected by the right relationships. The other premise is before a system can be redesigned it needs to be understood. Therefore, one purpose of the book is to broaden and deepen the readers' understanding of the structure of the U.S. healthcare system and the external forces that affect it. Another is to drill down to expose the mental models, which are the root causes of its undesirable events—inefficiencies, ineffectiveness, and inequities and show these events are tightly interdependent. The third purpose is to explain alternatives to the structure of the U.S. healthcare system and why some form of universal healthcare is the only *systemic* solution. The final purpose of this book is to give the reader hope that a healthier system is possible. By understanding the problems well enough, readers won't be misled by fear and gaslighting but can advocate for a systemic solution.

To accomplish this, the book uses the Iceberg Model (Figure 0.1) of systems thinking. Systems thinking is a diagnostic tool. It's way of perceiving our world in terms of

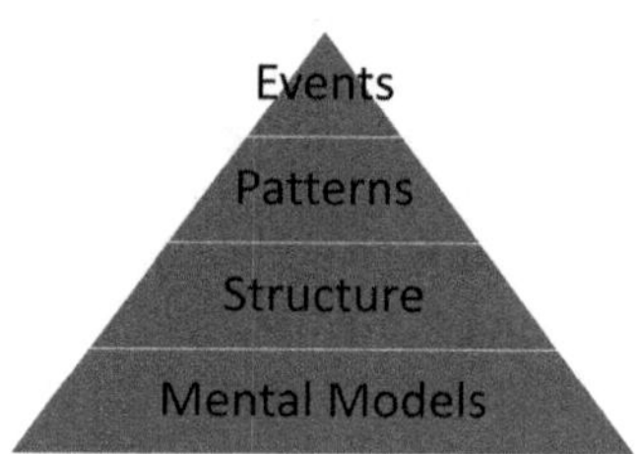


*Figure 0.1* Iceberg Model of Systems Thinking

wholes and relationships instead of separate, independent parts. *Events* refer to specific desirable and undesirable occurrences, such as last month's expenses, the number of new cases, and so forth. Events are what we see; they are above the water line. *Patterns* are the trends of events that occur over time. *Structure* refers to the organization of the system's parts. A system's structure generates the patterns and events. *Mental models* are beliefs and assumptions about our world. Because they inform, or generate, the structure of the system, they are often the root cause of undesirable events.

## Organization

This book is divided into three broad sections. The first section compares U.S. metrics for cost, quality, and equity with peer countries' metrics and explains why peer countries' costs, health outcomes, access, and equity are so much better than ours. As a reminder that healthcare is a complex *whole*, the section shows that cost, quality, and access—or efficiency, effectiveness, and equity—are interdependent. That is, to change one is to affect the other two. This section also shows the accrued effects of sixty years of piecemeal cost cutting activities are higher costs and explains why piecemeal reform has and will never work.

The second section offers two assumptions. One is the current U.S. healthcare system is out of date, and the other is we expect the U.S. healthcare system to do more than it was designed to do. Today's healthcare system arose with classical physics and chemistry, and the belief that the mind was separate from the body. Then, infectious diseases and trauma were the leading causes of death, and people didn't live as long. However, chronic diseases are the leading cause of death and disability today, and mental health issues are on the rise. Today, it's known healthcare determines about 10% to 20% of a person's health status; the other 80% to 90% is determined by the *social determinants of health.* These include such things as a safe and clean environment, affordable housing, and access to healthy foods, good education, and jobs. These are outside the healthcare system's control. When these social determinants are in short supply, people become chronically stressed, which leads to chronic diseases. One reason why peer countries have better health outcomes and healthier citizens is because of their "healthier" social policies and stronger social safety net.

The third section explains why relationships matter. Personally, social bonds are the number one source of good physical and mental health. Systemically, social bonds are the glue—the reinforcing and balancing feedback loops—that hold social systems and communities together. This section reminds the reader social systems are inspired by human thought, animated by human hands, and maintained by human habit. Because the healthcare system can never be better than the relationships of its stakeholders, this section reminds the reader it takes courage and compassion to overcome long-standing thoughts and habits and let go of old rules, roles, values, beliefs, and ideology, which stakeholders currently hold dear but exacerbate the current chaos.

Examining the healthcare through the lens of systems thinking, this book is intended to be a careful sorting out of the U.S. healthcare system and of the thought that generates it. It's an attempt to bring some order and understanding to the morass of contentious and confusing economic, moral, and political issues now perturbing the healthcare system. Readers will soon discover that I believe the U.S. healthcare system needs to be redesigned—that to create a new structure that is efficient, effective, equitable, and produces its intended product is to have some form of universal healthcare. It's a bold move, but, internationally, it's the only one that has been proven to work. The system we have now doesn't work well for anyone, except, perhaps, the financiers.

Believing that the only person anyone can change is one's self, the book invites readers to explore their own beliefs and values. Thus, at the end of each chapter are questions for the readers. They are starting points for the readers' own investigation into the challenges and possibilities for redesigning the structure of the U.S. healthcare system. More than anything, I hope readers will ask themselves the deepest question they can ask: What does it mean to care for other human beings? What is my responsibility to the whole?

As I write, I'm beginning my fiftieth year in healthcare. I started as a clinical dietitian and will close this journey as president of a small, rural hospital's board of trustees. It's definitely been an interesting and rewarding experience. Fifty years is a long time to be part of a social institution that is vital to the well-being of every American. Fifty years is also a long time to watch healthcare adapt, not always improve. It's a good time to advocate for a healthier healthcare system, one that works for everyone.

## Notes

1 Wager, E., McGough, M., Rakshit, S., Amen, K., & Cox, C. (January 23, 2024). How does health care spending in the US compare to other countries? Peterson-KFF Health System Tracker. https://www.healthsystemtracker.org/chart-collection/u-s-spending.

2 Amadeo, K. (October 21, 2022). The rising costs of health care by year and its causes. The Balance. https://www.thebalancemoney.com/causes-of-rising.

# 1 Review of Systems

## The Construction of the U.S. Healthcare System

### Current Reality

The COVID-19 pandemic was a shock to the U.S. healthcare system. It widened decades old fractures and added a few new ones, especially the distrust of science. Although the crisis is behind us, the optimism that healthcare would bounce back to "normal" has faded, replaced by dissatisfaction and worry. Very few Americans are happy with the U.S. healthcare system. According to a 2023 fourth quarter Keckley poll, "69% of [respondents] think the system is fundamentally flawed and in need of a major change, vs 7% who think otherwise; 60% believe it puts profits over people; and 74% think price controls are needed vs 7 who disagree."[1]

Today, the healthcare system doesn't work well for its primary stakeholders. If you're a patient, healthcare costs too much; wait times for appointments are too long; your insurance coverage is confusing and doesn't always cover what your doctor ordered; prescription drugs cost too much; and outcomes are not always good. If you are a doctor or a nurse, you're burned out; you're worried about your own safety because workplace violence is a daily reality; and your work-life balance feels, well, out of balance. If you're an independent hospital, your margins are paper thin; rising drug prices, staffing crisis, and inflation have bumped up costs; reimbursement doesn't always cover the cost of care; and insurers are getting better at denying, delaying, and disputing reimbursement.

### Unhealthy Systems Amplify Perturbations

Healthy systems are stable and stable systems are difficult to perturb. Stability implies a state of equilibrium, which is a kind of shock absorber. Because stable systems absorb, or dampen, internal and external chaos, they are difficult to perturb. In contrast, unhealthy systems are not at equilibrium. They are unstable and easy to perturb. Lacking shock absorbers, unstable systems amplify external shocks, which makes them even more unstable. Pushed too far, systems reach their tipping point where even a small perturbation can have deleterious consequences. In short, an unhealthy system is difficult to control and its future actions are less predictable than are that of a healthy system.

DOI: 10.4324/9781003538226-2

COVID-19, which revealed and exacerbated longstanding problems inherent in the U.S. healthcare system, further destabilized a system that was already teetering on the edge. COVID-19 triggered, or exacerbated, six interdependent, environmental perturbations. They are (1) physician and nurse burnout and worker shortages; (2) widespread and serious health inequities among the poor and people of color; (3) a growing mental health crisis; (4) the politicalization of healthcare and the loss of trust in science; (5) the marginalization of public health; and (6) new players disrupting the market, such as Amazon and CVS, UnitedHealth Group, respectively. COVID-19 also deepened the fracture lines between the system's primary parts: patients, doctors and hospitals, and insurers.

Even before COVID-19, the U.S. healthcare system was more expensive and had poorer health outcomes compared with other wealthy countries. The pandemic merely made things worse. For instance, in the winter of 2024, 50% of all rural hospitals—where 20% of Americans receive care—were operating in the red, and the outlook wasn't optimistic. All crisis are inflection points. That is, the situation either gets worse or better. To get worse means the structure of the system falls apart. To get better means evolution, or the synthesis of a novel and more complex system. For healthcare, evolution means healing fracture lines and integrating competitive parts into a more complex *whole.*

Healthcare is at an inflection point. We can choose to succumb to fear and continue to make piecemeal reforms, hoping to improve access for some, more affordability for others, and applying new layers of bureaucracy everywhere—all of which have brought us to today's inflection point. Or, we can choose to learn from the past; find the courage to remove our blindfolds and see the actual elephant that we're only partially aware of; and embrace novel thinking and bold systemic solutions. As Einstein stated, "Today's problems can't be solved with yesterday's thinking."

According to Jonas and Adibe, the challenge before us is:

> The current model of health care delivery has contributed to a relentless rise in medical costs, widening health disparities, growing dissatisfaction of patients, and burnout among clinicians. The COVID-19 pandemic has further exacerbated these long-standing challenges, highlighting the increasing need for social and mental health services. We need to fundamentally *redesign* (italics added) how care is provided so we can create health at lower cost.[2]

## The Blind Men and the Elephant

Americans' perspective of the U.S. healthcare system is much like the fable of the blind men and the elephant. The lesson of this story is that each blind man understood the elephant according to what he "saw," and each man was absolutely positive that the elephant was *the* part he was touching.

We understand what we see. In healthcare, the six stakeholder groups—(1) patients; (2) providers (doctors and hospitals); (3) payers (health insurance companies); (4) purchasers (businesses who subsidize health insurance for their employees); (5) purveyors (pharmaceuticals, etc.); and (6) politicians—are like the blind men and the elephant. Since each stakeholder group performs a different function, has different education and experiences, and expects different outcomes, it's not surprising each group has a different mental image of healthcare. Working in isolation, and trained and rewarded for protecting its competitive advantage, none of the stakeholders can imagine what the others perceive and experience.

The fable is a metaphor for the past sixty years of healthcare reform, efforts that resulted in higher costs, poorer health outcomes, and greater health disparities, compared with other wealthy countries. Each stakeholder group is partly right, but is totally wrong in believing that its version describes the whole healthcare system. The fable serves as a warning about being closed minded and advocating for a position based on a partial understanding of the system. Healthcare is too complex and too specialized for any one group to have all the answers. The fable is a statement that the whole cannot be reduced to its parts.

### What We See Determines What We Do

Despite the familiarity of the blind men and elephant metaphor, habits are hard to break. As a society, Americans tend to see problems in terms of "events" not "structures," and to reduce the problem to a broken part. In other words, we tend to "see" in terms of parts not wholes. This has led to intervening where the problem is most visible, such as legislation to reduce costs on ten drugs for the benefit of seniors while ignoring the fact that Americans pay about twice as much for pharmaceutical drugs than do citizens of other wealthy countries. For sixty years, access and cost have been perennial complaints and multiple fixes have been made, which have resulted in system heavily ladened with regulations and patchwork fixes. Yet, for sixty years, costs have continued to rise while access waxes and wanes.

To complicate matters, healthcare's visible problems differ depending whether one is a doctor, an employer, a patient, or an insurer. Thus, it's understandable that an employer would choose high-deductible insurance. That way he's "fixed" his high health insurance cost and continues to provide health insurance as an employee benefit. However, the effects of high-deductible insurance cascade through the system: Although the employers' costs go down, high-deductible insurance increases the employees' out-of-pocket costs. As more employees can't pay their out-of-pocket costs, hospitals have more bad debt. To compensate, hospitals raise their rates, which insurers then pass on to employers. And, the vicious cycle is complete. Being metaphorically blindfolded, it makes sense for stakeholders to optimize their part in the system without understanding their impact on the other stakeholders. Yet, vicious cycles end up being destructive, systemic perturbations.

### Seeing the Whole

Because what we see determines what we do, this book is about seeing the whole. If America is to escape the liabilities of piecemeal healthcare reform, which is guaranteed to further perturb an already unhealthy system, then we need to see the whole. By seeing the whole, we understand that the perennial concerns about affordability, access, quality, and equity of care are tightly inter-related and are the result of the system's structure. Once able to see the entire structure, we understand to change one undesirable event automatically affects other parts of the system, for good or ill. Because social systems are human constructs, created from human thought and animated by human hands, at a more abstract level, seeing the whole also refers to "seeing" the thought—the beliefs and values from which healthcare is formed.

If we continue with piecemeal reform, the result will be more of the same as sixty years of cost reduction "fixes" have shown. To paraphrase Albert Einstein, to do the same thing over and over but expect different results is insanity. Other experts put it this way: every system is perfectly designed to get the results it gets. To reiterate, for the U.S. healthcare system to provide care at a lower cost and improve access and health outcomes, then the solution is to redesign the structure of the healthcare system.

## Systems Thinking[3]

Systems thinking is a way for stakeholders to take off their blindfolds and see the whole elephant. Systems thinking is a conceptual framework that lets us see wholes rather than parts. Just as a person is can't be reduced to his organs, systems thinking is based on the theory that the whole is more than the sum of the parts. It's a shift from reductionistic thinking, which looks for "bad" people and "broken" parts, to a framework for evaluating the dynamic effect the interdependent parts have upon each other.

Systems thinking posits that a system's behavior is best understood by the virtue of the complex interdependent *relationships* among the elements that generate the system and the processes inside the system that generate its product. In other words, the product can never be better than the system that produces it and the functionality of a system can never be better than its parts and the relationships among the parts. To say it more bluntly, every social system is perfectly designed, by human beings, to get the results it gets.

## Hallmarks of a Healthy System Vis-à-Vis Flood's Holistic Prism

Robert L. Flood,[4] a leader in systems thinking, provides another way to see, understand, and evaluate systems. Briefly, Flood likens complex systems to a four-sided prism. Depicted in Figure 1.1, each of the prism's four facets reflects one aspect of the system: meaning, effectiveness, efficiency, and fairness.

Briefly, meaning has to do with purpose. The purpose of the healthcare system is to produce healthy people. Healthy systems produce their expected product. That the U.S. healthcare system does a better job producing profits than health indicates it doesn't fulfill its purpose. Effectiveness refers to whether the right parts are present so that the system can fulfill its purpose. The poorer health status of Americans indicates there are important, missing parts. (Effectiveness

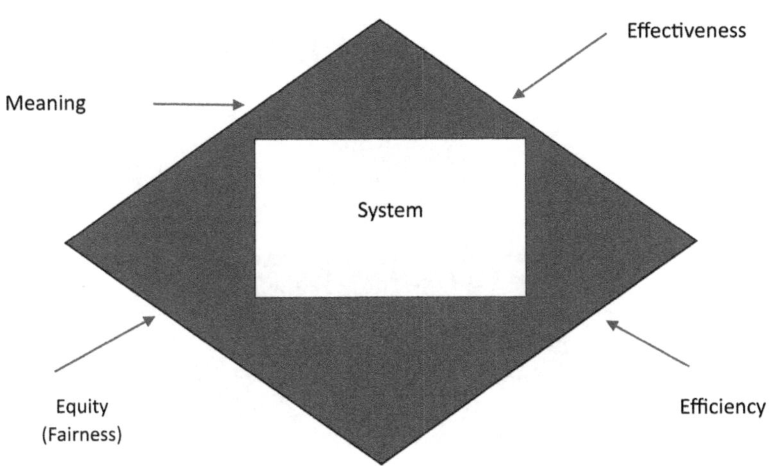


*Figure 1.1* Flood's Holistic Prism

is the subject of Chapters 6 and 7.) Efficiency refers to the conservation of resources. That America has the most expensive healthcare system in the world indicates that the U.S. healthcare system is inefficient. (Efficiency is the subject of Chapters 3–5.)

Fairness is a synonym for health equity. According to Flood, fairness refers to the ethical question of who is inside healthcare's boundaries and benefits and who is outside its boundaries and, therefore, loses. That the health status of the poor and people of color is worse than wealthier white people and access to healthcare is very difficult for people without health insurance indicate that the U.S. healthcare system is unfair. From Flood's perspective, fairness is obtained when the people drawing the system's boundaries choose for everyone the same as they choose for themselves and friends. That the poor and people of color have trouble accessing healthcare and tend to have poorer health status than wealthier white people indicate the U.S. healthcare system is not fair. (Fairness, or equity, is the subject of Chapters 7 and 8.)

## The Iceberg Model of Systems Thinking

The Iceberg Model is from Donella Meadows, a leader in systems thinking. The model is a diagnostic tool with four levels of analysis. By looking below the waterline, we can examine problems more thoroughly and accurately prior to acting. By moving from the superficial to the complex, each lower level offers a more thorough understanding of the interdependent interactions among the system's parts. Each level has its own leverage for change, with leverage increasing as the levels drop to the bottom of the iceberg. Instead of reacting to the most visible undesirable event at the tip of the iceberg, by revealing the root causes of *systemic* failures, the

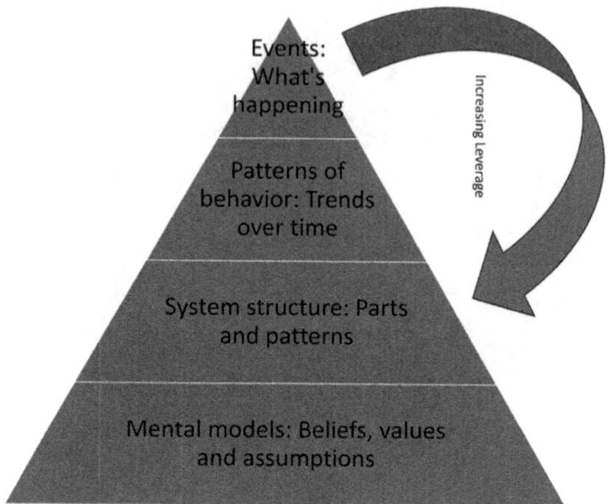


*Figure 1.2* Iceberg Model

model promotes acting from the place of greatest leverage, or greatest opportunity for *systemic* improvement (Figure 1.2).

**Events**

The events level provides data for "what's happening." Above the waterline, events are all that's visible. Analogous to symptoms in a medical diagnosis, events are measurable data, such as patient satisfaction surveys, the number of uninsured, access, geographic distribution of services, morbidity and mortality, health disparities, and so forth. Events show how the system is performing. Because events are generated by the structure of a system, events indicate the structure's soundness or healthiness. Using Flood's criteria, healthy healthcare systems are (1) efficient, they don't waste resources; (2) effective; their health outcomes are good; (3) equitable; everyone's included; and (4) they fulfill their purpose; they improve the health of individuals and communities. Local, national, and international data are used to evaluate the system's performance.

**Patterns**

The patterns of behavior level provide information about what's happening over time. Was the event a one-off; are the data getting worse or better over time? Is the pattern recurring, if so, under what conditions? Have we reached the threshold where we need to intervene? Patterns help with forecasting and forestalling events.

Patterns point to structure. Patterns show the performance of the structure over time and under changing conditions. Patterns raise questions about the soundness of the structure. Does the system have the right parts, are the boundaries the right size, and do the feedback loops function as they should? What's missing? Are the reinforcing feedback loops not balanced and out of control? This level indicates where systemic changes should be made.

## Structure

A system is a set of interconnected parts that are contained within a defined boundary and act according to a set of rules to produce a distinct product. Generally speaking, poor performance arises from structural problems: (1) the wrong set of parts; (2) boundaries that are too inclusive or exclusive; and (3) ineffective relationships among the parts. Thus, to improve a system's performance is to redesign its structure.

In systems thinking jargon, relationships are called feedback loops. Feedback loops are like a web that holds the parts together. Feedback loops carry information and resources among and between the parts. The two kinds of feedback loops—reinforcing and balancing—function like the gas pedal and brakes of a car, respectively. Reinforcing loops are the drivers of growth and decline; whereas, balancing loops are stabilizers, keeping the system at a desired level of performance. Together, they control the system's dynamic behavior.

Ideally, the right parts, in the right order, inside the right boundaries, with the right flow of information and resources between and among the parts results in a healthy system. To improve a system's performance is to redesign its structure.

## Mental Models

At the bottom of the iceberg lie the mental models. These are the accretion of thoughts—the beliefs, values, and assumptions—from which social systems, like healthcare, have evolved and the habits that maintain them. Generally speaking, mental models are so taken for granted that they are invisible and so habitual that we are not aware of their influence. That is—until they begin to fail. A sharp rise in the number of unexpected events and exceptions to the rule are sure signs of failing mental models. Lasting multiple unexpected events and exceptions to the rule raise issues not resolvable within the constraints of the prevailing mental model. Because of the accelerated pace of change, a mental model sows the seeds of its own destruction.

According to systems thinking, the root cause of every intractable systemic problem is either flawed or outmoded thinking, or the wrong purpose. Interventions at the root cause, or at the mental model level, have the greatest chance resolving the problems. However, mental models are very resistant to change. That is because we literally embody our mental models. They prescribe the way we learn to identify ourselves and embody that identity. Mental models inform our behavior, shape our social and civic relationships, and define our values and beliefs, including beliefs about sickness, health, and death, as well as beliefs about people not like us. Mental models even inform our beliefs about science.

The gift of the Iceberg Model is that it requires people to examine the decades of thinking from which a system has evolved, as well as their own thinking that maintains the current system. Because these thoughts are so deeply ingrained into our consciousness and so taken for granted, they are invisible until we deliberately bring them to light. For instance, Americans unquestionably accept the arbitrary linkage between health insurance and employment, accept universal health insurance as anathema, and then are surprised when tinkering with healthcare costs doesn't bring down costs but results in narrower networks and surprise billing.

Like the analogy of blind men and elephant, surfacing a system's mental models takes all its stakeholders. Because, like the blindmen, each of healthcare's stakeholder group belongs to a different part of the complex system and performs its own unique activities, no stakeholder group can see the whole without the insights of the others. For instance, legislators and policy analysts, physicians, insurance executives, and patients do not see the same thing. Neither do they have the same training nor have the same goals. Because of this uniqueness, each group experiences its own patterns and undesirable events. Therefore, each has its own solutions. Ineluctably, effective leverage comes from all of the stakeholder groups seeing and understanding all the four levels that represent the *whole* system. The fly in this ointment is for healthcare to change, each stakeholder group needs to change as well.

**The Basic Structure of Healthcare**

Like all systems, the U.S. healthcare system has a definable structure. It has definable boundaries; is composed of identifiable parts that are connected by networks of interlocking relationships; and produces a specific product, in this case, health (Figure 1.3).

The basic structure of every healthcare system has four parts: the patient, the healer, the cause(s) of disease, and the sanctioned treatment. The product, of course, is health. This is the basic structure, regardless of how primitive or sophisticated we deem a society's healthcare system.

Content varies according to society's understanding of the human body and its science and technology. The cause of disease(s) and sanctioned treatment vary according to society's understanding of the body and its science and technology, which is why, even today, a Navajo shaman, an allopathic physician, and a Traditional Chinese Medicine physician each sees different symptoms and recommends different treatments, even though they are looking at the very same patient.

The content also varies according to the moral value ascribed to sickness, the qualifications of its healers, and society's definition of health. Regardless of the model, patients are granted specific rights and benefits and have certain obligations to society. Patients may lose these rights and benefits, if they are not sick in the right way, such as being labeled neurotic or a maligner, or if the disease is stigmatized. This is especially true if the disease is contagious or is considered socially or morally wrong. Leprosy, HIV, and mental illness are examples of diseases associated with stigmas. Healers, likewise, have certain rights, privileges, and responsibilities.

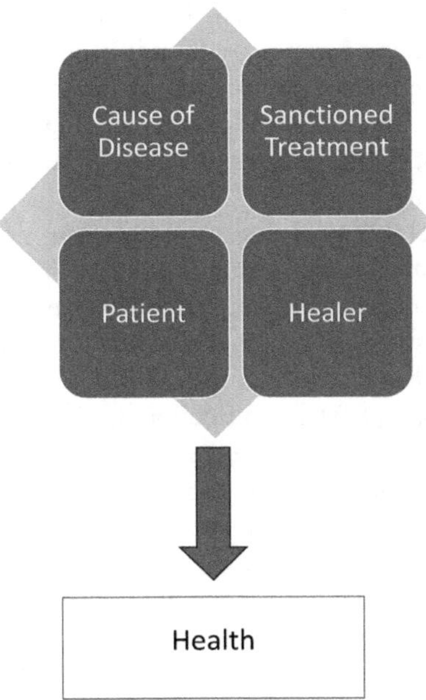


*Figure 1.3* Basic Structure of Healthcare

## Structure of the U.S. Healthcare System

Renowned for his work on healthcare history and policy, Paul Starr places the ascendency of our medical system between 1850 and 1930, a period Starr refers to as "medicine's civil war and reconstruction."[5] During this period, physicians pushed hard to establish the healthcare system on a firm scientific foundation. As a result, the core structure of the U.S. healthcare system is rooted in mental models associated with classical physics and chemistry, which presume a reductionistic, materialistic view of human beings and life itself (Figure 1.4).

In accordance with the knowledge and technology of the time, the U.S. healthcare system emerged from the time when people died from infectious diseases and work-related accidents. Then, antibiotics and childhood vaccines hadn't yet been invented. The mind was considered separate from the body; mental health was not healthcare's concern. The social determinants of health hadn't been discovered. Lives were too short for chronic diseases to be common or rehabilitation facilities,

| **Cause** | **Treatment** | **Health** |
|---|---|---|
| Biological pathology | Drugs & surgery | Absence of disease |
| **Patient** | **Healer** | |
| Person with biological pathology | Licensed physician | |

*Figure 1.4* Structure of U.S. Healthcare System

nursing homes and hospices to be need. Hospitals hadn't become "the doctors' workshops," since lifesaving technology hadn't been invented. The surgeries and drugs we take for granted today—joint replacement, organ transplantation, in vitro fertilization, immunotherapy drugs for cancer, etc.—were far beyond the horizon of anyone's imagination. Health insurance was very rare; costs were low; and people paid at the time of care.

Having its roots in classical physics and chemistry, the American healthcare system is based on the nineteenth-century definition of medicine: "the *science* of diagnosing, treating, and curing disease." Health is defined as the absence of disease. Because of their scientific training and licensing laws, physicians are the healer, to whom society has given the responsibility for producing health. Diseases are reduced to a biological problem—infection, toxins, trauma, faulty genes—and medical treatment is limited to drugs, surgery, and biotechnology.

Although other clinicians, such as chiropractors, nurse practitioners, and so forth, are often intimately involved in the treatment of a patient, doctors of medicine and osteopathy are acknowledged as the sole proprietors of the scientific knowledge and training needed to diagnose and treat disease. This proprietary knowledge gives physicians the authority to decide who is well and who is sick, which makes physicians gatekeepers to healthcare's services, as well as economic and social benefits, such as worker's compensation and social security disability benefits.

Patients are those the physician attests to as sick; that is, they have a demonstrable, biological pathology. This gives patients access to healthcare and permission to be excused from their regular family, civic, and economic responsibilities. However, if the patient is not sick in the correct way, he is a hypochondriac, for instance patients with fibromyalgia. If he has a stigmatized disease, such as substance abuse or HIV, he is blamed for his condition. If he seems to be taking financial or other advantage of his sickness, he is a malinger, such as a worker with chronic back pain. And, if he doesn't get well, he's labeled neurotic, which can happen to patients with rare or hard to diagnose diseases, such as Potts or Lyme disease. Any one of these conditions can disqualify a patient from access to healthcare and/or society's resources.

For a very long time, this construction of the U.S. healthcare system was remarkably stable and resistant to change. Because, for a very long time, healthcare was a cottage industry, meaning it was primarily composed of small, independent, local doctors and hospitals. Care was basically affordable and hospitals were a place where people went to die. However, once Medicare entered the market, the explosion of lifesaving drugs and technology took off and patients became consumers, the system began losing its resiliency. In 1964 healthcare represented only 5% of the GDP.

## In the U.S. Health Insurance Fractures Not Unites

The function of health insurance is the major difference between the U.S. healthcare system and that of other wealthy countries. In other wealthy countries, their doctors are licensed, similar to ours; their diagnoses and treatments of the sick are the same as ours; and they both use the same or similar technology. In other words, the core structure of their healthcare systems is identical to ours. The difference is the boundaries of their structure have been expanded to include health insurance as a part of their healthcare systems. It doesn't matter whether their health insurance is all private, all public, or a combination of both. At the end of the day, other wealthy systems, basically, have one funding stream. Hardwired into their healthcare systems, this one funding stream unites and delivers economic resources to all the parts of the healthcare system, much like blood flowing through the vascular system unites and delivers nutrients to all parts of the body.

In contrast, the U.S. has not hardwired the flow of funding into the structure of its healthcare system. Funding has always been bolted on, or external to the system. In fact, arbitrarily using the very early 1900s as a significant construction period, a major fault line was deliberately designed into its funding with the separation of public health and private medicine. According to Grogan,

> [t]he opposition was not against all forms of state activity; rather, they [private practice physicians] were primarily opposed to various forms of public insurance, compulsory insurance, and any expansion of public facilities to provide treatment beyond the indigent. However, because these physicians did support publicly funded treatment for indigents, where to draw the line—between the poor and non-poor or the needy and non-needy—was from a medical perspective, always ambiguous.[6]

Adding to the chaos, the U.S. has multiple payment systems: employer-subsidized insurance for most workers; traditional Medicare for some seniors; Medicare Advantage for other seniors; Medicaid for the qualified poor; VA benefits for veterans; and Workers' Compensation for injured workers. Despite six different payment systems, about 8% of Americans don't have health insurance. Moreover, six different payment systems and their six different sets of rules regarding which diseases and treatments will be covered fragment—not unite—the American system. The five sets of insurers, each in its own way, have usurped some of the clinical autonomy of American doctors. The scrutinizing of every test and every treatment the physician orders to avoid paying for care is harmful. It's the physician who knows the patient's needs, not the insurance company. It's the physician who has vowed to, "first do no harm," not the insurance company. The loss of clinical autonomy causes moral injuries to physicians and degrades the patient/physician relationship.

## Healthcare Is a Part and a Whole

Like all social systems, the healthcare system is both a part and a whole. Healthcare is not an independent system. It doesn't exist in a vacuum but is a system within a nested hierarchy of systems. Healthcare is enveloped by economic and social policies, and cultural values, which, in turn, are enveloped by the overarching mental models. In other words, to heal a fractured healthcare system, is to redesign the structure of healthcare itself.

This book is about seeing the whole healthcare system; it's also about the process of taking off our blindfolds. On one level taking off our blindfolds is to accurately

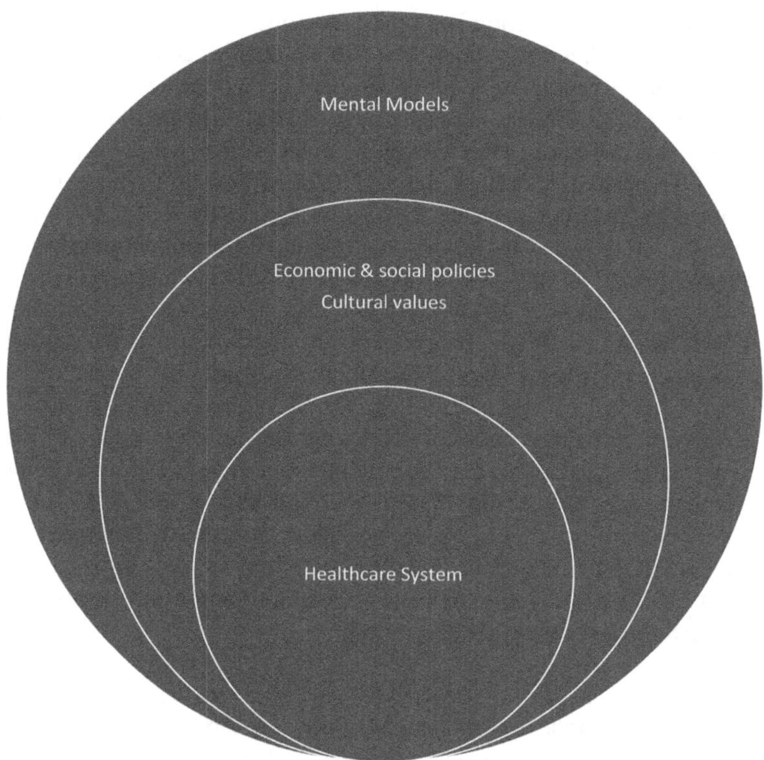


*Figure 1.5* Healthcare Is a Part and a Whole

see healthcare's current structure. This is a primary requirement necessary to design a system whose performance is efficient, effective, and fair. At a more abstract level, taking off our blindfolds is to expose and question our own mental models about the current structure and why and how the structure should be redesigned (Figure 1.5).

To effect true healing, both levels are important. Like the blindmen, each of healthcare's stakeholder group belongs to a different part of the complex system and performs its own unique activities; therefore, no stakeholder group can see the whole without the insights of the others. For instance, legislators and policy analysts, physicians, insurance executives, and patients do not see the same thing. They do not have the same training nor have the same needs, which in a healthy system are harmoniously balanced. Because of this uniqueness, each group experiences its own undesirable events and patterns, and, therefore, each has its own solutions.

Taking off our blindfolds also refers to escaping the blinders of fear, ignorance, and selfishness, which have been long-standing impediments to structural redesign. It's seeing each other as human beings, who have more in common than not, and finding compassion and restoring trust. Finally, taking our blindfolds off is about finding a shared vision of the desired future that each stakeholder group agrees and identifies with.

## U.S. Healthcare System Redux

America spends almost twice as much money on healthcare compared with similar wealthy countries, yet has the lowest life expectancy, highest burden of chronic disease, and the highest infant mortality rate. Knowledge about disease causation and treatment has evolved from healthcare's nineteenth-century linear production model and the germ theory of disease. However, it's well documented chronic diseases, the leading causes of death and disability today, are caused by complex interactions of social, economic, and environmental factors, which under the right conditions can lead to biological pathology. Plus, the need for mental health services continues to grow. However, physicians still have the sole responsibility for producing health using drugs and surgery (Figure 1.6).

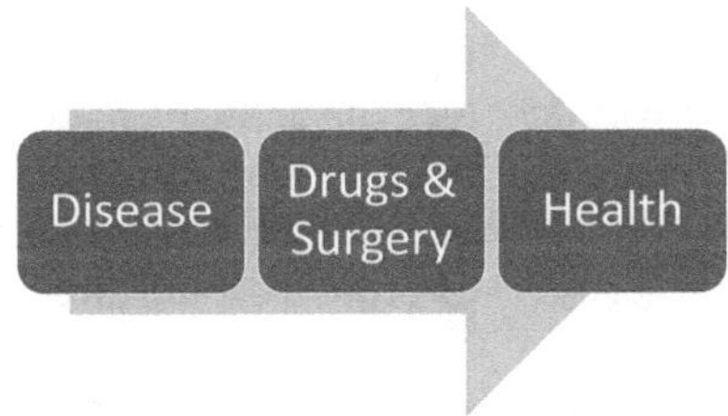


*Figure 1.6* Linear Production Model

It's also well documented that patients want healthcare that is affordable, easy to access, timely, convenient, and personalized, or to use the jargon, patient-centered. Since COVID-19, physicians want a less stressful system. They want more autonomy, greater control over the practice of medicine, fewer hassles from insurance companies, student loan repayment, and better work-life balance. Nurses want to feel safe, appreciated, and adequately compensated. Finally, hospitals want enough staffing to provide safe, quality care and a large enough margin to stay in business. Today, these three vitally important providers are seriously perturbed.

Healthcare is something everyone needs. Sickness, frailty, and death are part of the human condition. No one wants to die alone or in pain. No one should be afraid to seek lifesaving care because they can't afford it. Jail is not "treatment" for the mentally ill and addicted. Healthcare is more than a social safety net; it is a reflection of how we care for each other.

## Questions for the Reader

The questions provide an opportunity to examine your own mental models and values and to imagine other stakeholders' beliefs, fears, and values.

1 What is the purpose of the U.S. healthcare system? Is it to produce healthy citizens or profits for investors? Do you believe it fulfills its purpose? Why do you believe this; what might others?
2 Is the current healthcare system unhealthy? What evidence do you have that supports your answer?

3 Which stakeholder group are you in? Are you a patient, a physician, a hospital, or representative? Does the healthcare system meet your needs? If yes, what needs are met? If no, what needs are not being met?
4 In your experience, is the current system is effective, that is, have you been satisfied with the outcome of treatment? Does America have the best—the most effective—healthcare system in the world? Why; what might others believe?
5 In your experience, does healthcare cost too much? Have you, or someone you know, not signed up for health insurance, delayed care, or not filled a prescription because of costs? If so, what was the result? Do you believe healthcare should be affordable for everyone? Or, should healthcare be available only to those who can afford the purchase price? Why; what might others believe?
6 In your experience, is the healthcare system fair? Have you, or someone you know, received care that wasn't so good because of race, gender, or socioeconomic status? How did that make you feel?
7 Do you know anyone who lost their insurance because they lost their job, got divorced, moved, or made too much money to qualify for Medicaid? Do you believe everyone should be treated equitably? Why; what might others believe?
8 Should everyone have access to affordable healthcare? Why; what might others believe?
9 What do you value about the current healthcare system? What do you not value or find problematic? What might others value or find problematic with the current system?

## Notes

1 Keckley Poll: The public is fed up with the U.S. health care system … so what else is new. (2023, November 20). *The Keckley Report.* www.paulkeckley.com/the-keckley-report/2023/11.
2 Jonas, W.B., & Adibe B. (2022, May 20). An integrated framework for achieving national health goals. *JAMA Network.* https://jamanetwork.com/journals/jama-health/forum/issue/3/5.
3 Stroh, D.P. (2015). *Systems Thinking for Social Change: A Practical Guide to Solving Complex Problems, Avoiding Unintended Consequences, and Achieving Lasting Results.* White River Junction, VT: Chelsea Green Publishing.
4 Flood, R.L. (1999). *Rethinking the Fifth Discipline: Learning within the Unknowable.* London and New York: Routledge. p. 70.
5 Starr, P. (1982). *The Social Transformation of American Medicine.* New York: Basic Books.
6 Grogan, C.M. (2023). *Grow and Hide: The History of America's Health Care State.* New York: Oxford University Press. p. 14.

# 2 Efficiency

## The Human Costs of Inefficiency

Efficiency is a measure of how well a system is performing. Efficiency is defined as the ability to achieve maximum output with minimum input. Efficiency is measured by the amount of resources—money, time, etc.—used to produce a product. In this case, efficiency refers to the amount of money the U.S. spends to produce healthy citizens. The U.S. healthcare system is notoriously expensive. In 2022, America spent an average of $12, 555 per person compared with the per person average $6,651 spent by its eleven peers—Germany, Switzerland, Netherlands, Austria, Sweden, France, Canada, Australia, the United Kingdom, Belgium, and Japan. Of the peer countries, Japan spent the least, an average of $5,251.[1]

Today, healthcare in the U.S. is a $4.5-trillion dollar enterprise. However, an increasing number of Americans find healthcare unaffordable. U.S. adults owe at least $195 billion in medical debt; about 40% of Americans have unpaid medical bills; and 38% don't seek needed healthcare because they can't afford it. Healthcare is the leading cause of household debt; 50% of the U.S. bankruptcies are caused by unpayable medical bills even though most of the families had health insurance. A little over 10% of adult Americans don't have health insurance. Another 43% of working-age adults are under insured, meaning they had a gap in coverage during the year or the cost of their deductibles, co-pays, and coinsurance are more than they can afford.[2]

## Where Does the Money Come From?

The $4.5 trillion the U.S. spends on healthcare comes from a combination of public and private monies. According to Grogan, "If we add up all the items that are funded through taxation, public taxpayers cover 60% of national health expenditures. While this level of public funding is substantial, it is seldom discussed or portrayed, and it is almost certainly more than sixty percent."[3] Of the remainder, private business and households, and philanthropy account for another 35% and 5%, respectively.[4] Of the private money, health insurance accounts for 31%, with about 48% of private sector employees having employer subsidized health insurance. Out-of-pocket expenses account for 12% and other third-party payers account for the remaining 11%.[5]

DOI: 10.4324/9781003538226-3

It's worth noting that households bear the ultimate burden of financing the U.S. healthcare system. The money comes from the out-of-pocket expenses for deductibles and co-pays, plus the household's share of the premium if they have employer-subsidized insurance or the cost of the premium if they are individually insured. Although an employee benefit, employer-subsidized health insurance isn't a gift. Employees pay. Hidden in the cost of health insurance is the cost of lost wages associated with employer premium subsidies, as well as Federal Insurance Contributions Act (FICA), state, and other taxes. Medicaid is a separate state tax which almost everyone pays. Americans pay for healthcare through the cost of their auto and home owners insurance, which include some coverage for medical expenses.

A painful paradox is that the uninsured wage earner subsidizes the insured. Every time he or she buys a car or other items the insured produce, the uninsured help subsidizes the coverage of the insured. Because health benefits are not taxed as income—for example an employer-paid benefit worth $500 a month is actually $6,000 in income that's not taxed—the uninsured loses twice.

Public monies fund the healthcare systems in Austria, Sweden, Netherlands, Canada, and Great Britain. These systems are paid for by some form of *progressive* tax, which, essentially, every household pays. On the other hand, the U.S., Japan, Germany, Switzerland, and Australia use a combination of private and public monies to fund their systems. Regardless of whether the money is public or a mix of public and private, peer countries pay less than half what the U.S. pays for healthcare and they have universal healthcare.

All of their citizens are covered, have the same covered benefits, and everyone has access to affordable care. However, different countries have different covered benefits. For example, dental care is a covered benefit in Japan, Germany, and Great Britain, but not covered in Canada and Switzerland. Nursing home care is a covered benefit in Germany, Austria, Japan, and Switzerland, but not in Canada. In contrast to the others, only Canada does not cover out-patient prescriptions drugs but does cover drugs administered during a hospitalization.

Because everyone is covered, people living in peer countries aren't burdened with narrow networks and surprise billing. For those living in peer countries, public and private costs are progressive, which is not the case for Americans. For example, in the U.S., a low-wage worker will pay proportionately more of his wages for health insurance than a high-wage earner, in the same company. Besides making care affordable for everyone, peer countries also standardize their covered benefits and cost-sharing formulas, whereas, in the U.S. both are left up to the numerous public and private insurers.

## Where Does the Money Go?

For decades, costs have steadily risen, yet where the money goes has been remarkably stable. The bulk of the money consistently goes to hospitals—about 31%. The other top receivers are physicians and clinical services at 20%; prescription drugs at 9%; and administrative costs at 7%. The remainder goes to services such as home care, nursing homes, durable medical equipment, dental, and so forth.[6]

It's tempting to attribute the U.S.'s remarkably expensive healthcare system to having more doctors, hospital beds, and better quality of care than peer countries. However, that is not the case, according to the KFF Health System Tracker.[7] On a per capita basis, the U.S. does not have nearly as many hospitals nor hospital beds as its peers. For example, the peer average is 4.2 beds per 1,000 population, with the U.S. at 2.5 beds per 1,000 population. Japan has the most, 7.8 beds per 1,000 population, and Sweden and Canada have the fewest, 2.0 beds per 1,000. The average length of hospital stay is shorter in American hospitals than in peer countries.

The U.S. has more nurses than most of its peers. For example, the peer average is 14.6 nurses per 1,000 populations, with the U.S. having 17.4 nurses and Sweden having the most at 20 nurses per 1,000. Among its peers, only Japan has fewer physicians per capita than the U.S., but have enough for the Japanese to see their doctors about thirteen times per year compared with four times a year for Americans. While peer countries have increased their supply of physicians since 2000, the U.S. has not, resulting in a physician shortage. The impact of physician shortage is felt nationwide. It's not uncommon for Americans, regardless of where they live, to wait two to six months for an appointment with a specialist. The physician shortage is worse for people living in sparsely populated rural areas. They are five times more likely than those living in urban and suburban areas to not have enough local doctors.

The U.S. spends more than its peers on expensive technologies, like MRI and robotic surgery, and more on expensive procedures, like Cesarean sections and joint replacement surgery. Prescription drugs cost about four times more in the U.S. Lastly, the U.S. healthcare system has more employees than its peers. About 14% of all U.S. workers are employed in healthcare, making it the largest U.S. employer.

Finally, the U.S. spends a lot more on administrative overhead than its peers—an average of $925 per person compared with the peer average of $204 per person.[8] Administrative costs refer to expenses such as marketing, customer service, billing and insurance related costs, executive salaries, and dividends paid to stockholders. In contrast to the U.S., peer systems do not have the expense of stockholder dividends, nor do they pay their physicians and executives as much as America does. Administrative costs vary widely in the U.S., ranging from about 2% for traditional Medicare to somewhere between 15% and 30% for private insurance.

## The U.S. Healthcare System Wastes Resources

Healthy systems are efficient. An efficient system uses its resources in the right way; it produces its product without wasting resources. The U.S. healthcare system is inefficient. While multiple studies have estimated that about 20% to 30% of healthcare spending is waste, a 2019 study reported in JAMA, which consolidated seven years of findings, estimated the U.S. healthcare system wastes $760 billion annually:[9]

- Care delivery—not doing the right thing or doing the wrong thing—wastes $102.8 billion
- Care coordination—fragmented care or patients falling through cracks in system—wastes $27.2 billion

- Overtreatment—unnecessary or low value care—wastes $75.5 billion
- Administrative complexity—billing and coding, and physician time spent on quality measures—wastes $265.6 billion
- Pricing failure—complexities and lack of transparency—wastes $230.7
- Fraud and abuse waste $58.5 billion

## Why the U.S. Pays More for Healthcare than Its Peers

Why does the U.S. pay almost twice as much for healthcare than its peers? It's a good question, since like almost all of its peers, the American system is a mix of public and private doctors and hospitals and public and private insurers. (The two exceptions are totally public Great Britain and totally private Switzerland.)

It can't be said often enough: Every system is perfectly designed to get the results it gets. So, what makes the U.S. system more costly with poorer health outcomes than Germany, Japan, or France—peer countries that also are a mix of public and private providers and insurers? The superficial reason is Americans pay more for healthcare is because its prices are much higher than its peers. The root cause, however, is found in its design. It's designed to have high prices. Among its peers, the U.S. is the only *for-profit* system. As with any for-profit business, each sector of healthcare—hospitals, pharmaceutical companies, physician groups, private (commercial) insurers, and so forth—expects its profits to grow quarterly. As a for-profit system, waste is baked into the design of the U.S. healthcare system. What one stakeholder group calls waste, others call profits.

## Global Budgets Control Costs

In contrast, peer countries' healthcare systems are efficient. Peer countries control their costs in two ways. First, healthcare in peer countries is non-profit. Since their stakeholders are not motivated by quarterly growth and increasing stockholder value, peer countries can keep their costs low. Second, peer countries have *one* healthcare system funded by a global budget. Global budgets are to healthcare systems as the blood supply is to the body. Both maintain the health of the whole. Just as the body's organs share a finite amount of blood, with a global budget, stakeholders share a finite amount of funds.

A global budget refers to the fixed, total amount of money that a country has available to spend on healthcare annually. Simply speaking, a global budget is funded through some form of progressive taxes, like Great Britain and Canada, or a combination of progressive taxes and limited household contributions, like Japan and Germany. Access is universal and costs are controlled. Price ceilings and expenditure caps allow for margins but control profits. Regulations are put in place to assure quality. Global budgets take into account factors such as geography so that sparsely populated rural areas can count on having healthcare. Just as the body can adjust the distribution of blood depending on need, global budgets allow for adjustments such as specifying the maximum amount of money spent by disease, the type of hospital or medical facility, and so forth. Simply speaking, a global budget means that healthcare dollars are invested in the health of the community and those who live there.

## Our Fragmented Funding "System"

Unlike its peers with their global budgets, the funding of the U.S. healthcare system is highly fragmented. Instead of one pool of money that covers everyone, the U.S. healthcare system is funded by a mix of public and private insurance monies. Public insurance is further fragmented into traditional Medicare for seniors; Medicaid for the qualified poor, blind and disabled, and destitute nursing home residents; CHIPS (Children's Health Insurance Program) for poor children; and the VA and Tricare for the military and their dependents. On the private, or commercial, side of the ledger are employer-subsidized private insurance, for many, but not all workers; individual private insurance for the self-employed; Medicare Advantage, a private insurance for seniors; and workers' compensation for people with qualified job-related injuries, although there are some federal compensation programs, such as the Black Lung Program for coal miners and their dependents. Adding to the fragmentation, private insurers are expected to return a percentage of their revenue to investors and stockholders.

It gets worse. The cost of private insurance is further fragmented by market size and geography. Thus, costs vary widely, according to whatever the market will bear. For instance, large employers, which have more leverage, get better rates than smaller employers and the self-employed. Mining, agriculture, and other employers for high-risk jobs pay more for health insurance than those who employ office workers. People living in sparsely populated states, like Wyoming, pay about twice what people living in Maryland pay for health insurance. Cost also varies by gender and age. Women of childbearing age pay more than men for the same policy, and younger adults pay more than adults between the ages of 55 and 64. Implicit in this fragmented funding system is each revenue stream should cover its own costs.

For small businesses, self-purchasers, and seniors wanting to supplement their Medicare, fragmentation makes shopping fraught. Although by law, Affordable Care Act (ACA) certified plans have the same ten basic elements of coverage, premiums vary widely, as do out-of-pocket costs. In one town, according to anecdotal evidence, premiums varied from $60 to $400 per month for a certified Medicare supplemental plan. Low monthly premiums don't always translate into cost saving, since low premiums are associated with higher co-pays, co-insurance, and deductibles. Generally speaking, low premiums are safe for people who are younger, in good health, and seldom use healthcare services. Because of fragmentation, not all plans have an out-of-pocket maximum, in other words, a cap on the person's annual out-of-pocket costs. And, different plans have different formularies, meaning that your plan may not cover the name brand of the drug you take but something your insurer considers comparable.

Because of our fragmented funding "system," access to healthcare is also fragmented. A global budget with concomitant universal access is salutary. Universal healthcare allows everyone access to medical care. Universal healthcare eliminates the risk of losing health benefits because of a change in address, employment, age, or health status. It eliminates the devastation of losing health benefits when one loses one's job—a stressful time that often compromises health. And, universal healthcare eliminates the emotional and financial stress of having to pay in advance for non-emergent surgeries and procedures, or having your physician refuse to care for you if you have an unpaid bill, a barrier to care that is becoming more common.

### The Lack of Standardization Is Costly to Hospitals

There are about 1,600 private insurers in the U.S. Each has multiple different plans with their own set of rules, regulations, and requirements, which change constantly. Generally speaking, none of them pay the same rate for the same procedure, with the exception of traditional Medicare. The result is expensive. Because of our complex funding mechanisms, Americans spend much more on billing than peer countries, accounting for about 30% of the waste in the U.S. healthcare system.[10] Devoid of standardization, efficiency is impossible.

The unifying factor of a global budget is all doctors and hospitals are paid the same amount for the same service, period. With our highly fractured system, payment varies radically, according to the patient's insurance. Because of the huge national variation in providers' prices and private insurers' reimbursement, comparison data are generalized. Generally speaking, traditional Medicare and Medicaid pay less than private insurance and the payment doesn't cover the cost of care. A KFF study reported private insurance pays 1.6–2.5 higher than Medicare pays for inpatient services; for out-patient services private insurers pay about 2.6 more than Medicare; and private insurance pays physicians about 1.4 higher than Medicare.[11] There's even more variation between Medicaid reimbursement and private insurance. As a combination of federal and state monies and regulation, each state determines how much Medicaid pays providers. In most states, Medicaid pays about 80% of Medicare; however, estimates show as much as a fivefold difference among the states.

### Cost Shifting

Global budgets with their same payment for the same service eliminate cost shifting. Cost shifting refers to hospitals and other providers making up for the lower payments from Medicare and Medicaid by charging private insurers more. Cost shifting is like the competitive children's game of musical chairs where the fastest and largest child typically wins. Unfortunately, cost shifting exacerbates system fragmentation and fragmentation exacerbates cost shifting.

### Profit Protection Is the Name of the Game

As with musical chairs no one wants to be the loser. To stay in the game, private insurers and hospitals—regardless of whether they are for-profit or non-profit—have engaged in several decades of profit-protecting adjustments. The differences between for-profit and non-profit hospitals are for-profit hospitals are investor owned and don't pay taxes, whereas, in lieu of taxes non-profit hospitals don't pay taxes but are supposed to provide a commensurate amount of uncompensated care to their communities.

Since size is protective, both hospitals and insurers continue to consolidate to gain economies of scale, market power, and leverage. Today, the top five health insurance companies control about 46% of the insurance market and the top fifteen large hospital systems control about a third of the hospital market. While economies of scale have benefited large insurers and hospital systems, the cost savings haven't been shared with patients.

Besides consolidation, hospitals typically protect their profits by raising rates, eliminating unprofitable services, and/or moving services to profitable locations. Emergency, obstetric, and pediatric services are often at risk for closure, especially if they have high volumes of uninsured and Medicaid patients. Due to financial pressures, over 400 maternity services closed between 2006 and 2020, and about half of rural areas don't have maternity services. From 2008 to 2018, 20% of in-patient pediatric units were closed, resulting in longer distances to care for about 25% of U.S. children. Some urban hospitals in low-income neighborhoods simply close their doors; others move to wealthier, better insured suburbs. Some large hospital systems offer their own insurance products, directly competing with insurance companies. Today, about 40% of large hospital systems offer insurance products, which gives them two revenue streams and better control over the utilization of services.

Aggressive collection practices are used by many hospitals. This can include taking patients to court, garnishing wages, placing liens on houses, and selling their bad debt to collection agencies. Some hospitals are offering medical credit cards, although with their high interest rates they are a poor product for most people. About 20% of hospitals deny non-emergent care to patients with unpaid balances, and some are asking the bill be paid in full *prior* to non-emergent surgery or other procedures. With about 18% of the U.S. and households having medical debt and about 80% of them having some form of insurance coverage, coverage wasn't adequate to protect them from the financial hardship caused by co-pays, deductibles, co-insurance costs, uncovered services, and/or network restrictions.[12]

Like hospitals, insurers also have multiple ways to protect their profits. The easiest ways are to raise rates on premiums, increase co-pays and deductible, and tighten provider networks. To do this they change their rules annually. An increasingly common profit-protecting move is prior authorization. This requires extra documentation and physician time that the test, drug, or procedure is necessary. The downside is that the annual rule changes create more inefficiencies in the provider sector. According to one report, 39% of physicians spend as much as one to nine hours per week petitioning insurers to pay for care their patients need. This waste of time ultimately raises healthcare costs. Prior authorization also unnecessarily delays care and often leads to poorer health outcomes.

Insurers also have a history of "cherry picking" and "lemon dropping." The cliché of the signup office on a third-floor walkup is well known example of cherry picking. Lemon dropping refers to excluding certain types of "expensive" providers from the insurer's network. This includes such things as avoiding hospitals that won't accept the discounted reimbursement rate and carving high-cost specialty physician groups out of the hospital's network. Insurers also protect their profits by not covering certain types of expensive services, such as in-vitro fertilization and cosmetic surgery and by keeping some high-cost drugs off their formularies. Some large insurers have expanded into others' markets. For instance, United Health now includes a large network of doctors, pharmacy benefit managers, and other services, which gives them multiple revenue streams and tight control over the utilization of medical care and pharmaceutical drugs.

The effects of these profit-protecting adjustments have been good for business. U.S. spending on healthcare rose from $1.4 trillion in 2000 to $4.5 trillion in 2023. The real losers, however, are the patients. Despite claims of reduced costs, research shows that consolidation in the insurance and hospital markets has resulted in higher prices in both markets than in unconsolidated markets. Although many hospitals have added financial navigators to help patients sign up for insurance and qualify for pharmaceutical and other financial resources, it's the patient and public who pay. Cost savings to insurers has not resulted in reduced premium costs to patients. Instead, premium costs rose annually between 2000 and 2022, a whopping 215% increase, compared with a cumulative inflation rate of 57%,[13] and out-of-pocket costs rose essentially the same percentage.[14]

### Cost-Shifting Redux

The fragmented design of the U.S. healthcare system enables the stronger stakeholder groups to protect their profits by shifting costs to the weaker group, that is, to the part least able to protect itself. Historically, this is the patient. More recently, however, there's another vulnerable group: small, rural hospitals. About 30% of rural hospitals are at risk of closure. Fifty percent of independent rural hospitals operated in the red during 2023, the largest percentage of rural hospitals losing money in the past decade.[15] They have been hit hard by the twin forces of rising costs and stagnant reimbursement. For many of these hospitals, private insurance and Medicare rates are too low to cover their costs of care. With approximately 20% of Americans receiving care from rural hospitals, their closure would be a significant loss, indeed.

Ultimately, everyone pays. Hospitals make up for uncompensated care by raising prices. Since Medicare and Medicaid payments are fixed, the higher prices are paid by the private insurers, which causes insurance companies to raise their rates and employers to shift more of the cost to employees, which means more people can't afford healthcare and more uncompensated care for hospitals and poorer health outcomes for people, which triggers the next round of the vicious cycle of raising prices.

### The Human Costs of Inefficiency

Peer countries have healthcare systems that are efficient. Their average cost per citizen is less than half what Americans pay, $6,125 versus $12,914, respectively. Peer countries control their costs through a global budget. There's no cost shifting because their systems are non-profit and include everyone under the same global budget. In contrast, the fragmented structure of the U.S. healthcare system ensures cost shifting, which ensures the elimination of the weakest stakeholders. Historically, this is the patient. More recently, however, small rural hospitals and safety net hospitals are at risk of closure. Safety net hospitals are urban hospitals that generally serve the elderly, Medicaid, and uninsured patients. By caring for the uninsured and under insured, safety net hospitals operate on tissue thin margins. Their very thin margins and few endowments make them vulnerable for closure.

In 2024, about 30% of rural hospitals are at risk of closure.

Two rural groups especially vulnerable to loss are cancer patients and pregnant women. Due to financial pressures, over 400 maternity services closed between 2006 and 2020 and half of rural areas have no maternity services. The loss of maternity service contributes to America having the highest infant and maternal mortality rates of wealthy nations. Between 2014 and 2022, financial pressures also pushed 47% of rural hospitals to stop providing chemotherapy services,[16] contributing to the increased likelihood of premature deaths.

Other especially vulnerable groups are low-income workers and the self-pay. To compensate for the ever-increasing health insurance premiums, employers increasingly use high-deductible health plans, shifting more of the costs to employees. A growing percentage of low-wage employees don't sign up for health insurance because they can't afford their share of the premium. Others sign up but go without routine care because they can't afford the typical $5,000 to $10,000 deductible. It's shocking that almost 40% of Americans *with* health insurance didn't seek medical care in 2021 because of fear of costs; 25% of women put off preventive care because of unaffordable out-of-pocket costs;[17] and 30% with health insurance didn't fill a needed prescription. While some low-income workers' wages are low enough to qualify for Medicaid, most either make too much to qualify or don't meet other qualifying criteria.

Painfully, the people who don't have health insurance but make too much to qualify for Medicaid end up paying the most for healthcare. Their care is not discounted. They pay the "sticker price," about 2.5 times more than what a group or individual plan would pay. The irony is that they pay twice: First, because they can't afford and don't have health insurance, they're billed the full price. Second, they subsidize everyone else's insurance through taxes and by buying the goods and services made by those who have employer-subsidized insurance.

Efficiency and effectiveness are tightly interrelated. Many of the uninsured also pay with their lives. Uninsured Americans generally die sicker and prematurely. Without insurance they don't receive preventative treatment. When sick they put off going to the doctor until the problem has reached an advanced stage where care is less effective and more expensive. When the problem becomes too great to manage at home, they go to the nearest emergency department for care where they are stabilized and referred to seek specialized care. Uninsured, they are left to navigate a system of safety-net services and charity care where options vary widely by region. There is very little data about the number who falls through the cracks. What is known is the uninsured die sicker and prematurely and this lack of access contributes to the moral injury of physicians and physician burnout.

The fragmented design of the U.S. healthcare system assures cost shifting and the risk of being excluded from healthcare. According to the design, the costs are shifted to the part least able to protect itself. Ironically, at the end, everyone pays. Hospitals make up for uncompensated care by raising prices. Since Medicare and Medicaid payments are fixed, the higher prices are paid by the private insurers. When rates are raised, employers shift more of the cost to employees, so more people can't afford healthcare. This leads to poorer health outcomes for people and more uncompensated care for hospitals. More uncompensated care triggers the next round of raising prices and poorer health outcomes. This vicious cycle shows efficiency and effectiveness are interrelated. To change one is to affect the other.

## Efficiency Is a Function of Purpose

Every system is perfectly designed to get the results it gets. A healthy system produces its expected product. In this case, the expected product is health. A healthy system is also efficient—it doesn't waste resources. Is the U.S. healthcare system efficient? The answer is, it depends on its purpose. If the purpose is to produce health, then based on health outcomes that aren't as good as peer countries and its much higher costs, the U.S. system is not efficient.

However, if the purpose is to produce wealth for some stakeholders, then the U.S. system is highly efficient. The system works very well for insurers. For instance, almost one out of four dollars flows through the big six insurance companies. In 2023, the three largest insurers—UnitedHealth Group, CVS Health, and Elevance Health—had a combined profit of $32.7 billion.[18] Likewise, the system works well for large hospital systems. The combined profits of the three largest hospital systems—HCA Healthcare, Kaiser Permanente, and Tenet Healthcare—were $10.6 billion in 2023.[19] Despite the positive post-COVID-19 profit margins, about 40% of U.S. hospitals are still losing money from operations in 2024.[20]

From a systemic perspective, the U.S. healthcare system is a $4.5-trillion industry, represents 18% of the GDP, and has 14.7 million direct employees, the most employees of any U.S. industry. Actually, the U.S. healthcare system is the fourth largest economy in the world, replacing Germany as number four.

## Costs Cannot Be Controlled in a Fragmented, For-Profit System

Despite 50 years of intermittent cost containment efforts, costs have continued to rise, representing 7% of the GDP in 1970 but 18% in 2022. Per capita costs also rose during this period, from $1,951 to $12,914. Costs cannot be controlled in a

Events:
High prices
Patterns: Ever rising prices
Structure: Fragmented funding stream
Mental Models: For profit, healthcare is a commodity

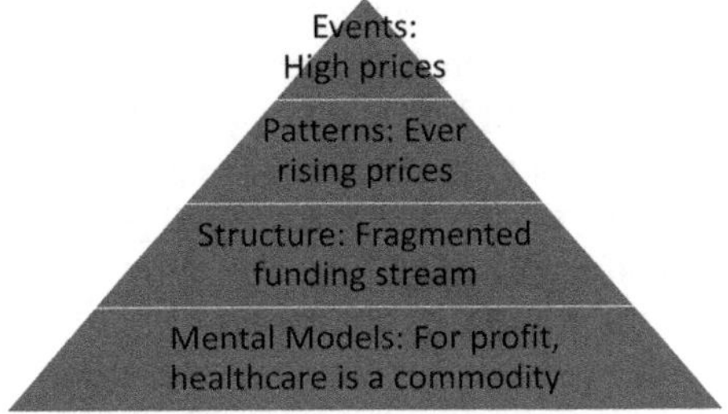

*Figure 2.1* Iceberg Model: Drivers of U.S. Healthcare Costs

fragmented system; they can only be shifted, typically to those who have the least political power to protect themselves. Despite good intentions and pragmatism, attempting to control rising costs through piecemeal reform will always fail. As Figure 2.1 shows the drivers of rising costs are a fragmented funding stream and for-profit mental models.

## Why the U.S. Keeps Its For-Profit Healthcare

To summarize, America has the most expensive healthcare system in the world, with costs rising annually. It's the only system in the developed world that doesn't cover everyone. It's the only system in the developed world that is for-profit. Despite its high costs, the U.S. healthcare system's access, health outcomes, and equity are second tier compared to peer countries.

Since World War II, either Congress or a president has periodically advocated for some form of universal healthcare. From a systems thinking perspective, the root causes of these failures are the mental models that inform the system. Mental models are the various beliefs, values, and assumptions that maintain America's for-profit system.

Because the influence of mental models is significant, it's worth investigating the most common beliefs and values for their validity. For starters, distrust of the government and fear of "socialized medicine" are the most common reasons used against universal healthcare. However, seniors like their traditional Medicare and its administrative costs are significantly less than private insurance. Similarly, universal healthcare is frequently equated with socialized medicine; however, the Swiss system is fully privatized and the Germans have a mix of public and private. The Swiss system is regulated by the federal government and the German system is regulated by a quasi-private board. Both countries have lower costs and better health outcomes than the U.S.

Another common reason is universal healthcare will cost more, but decades of comparison costs prove otherwise. Americans pay about twice what citizens of peer countries pay. A similar claim that universal healthcare will inexorably raise taxes is also false, considering the average family premium of $22,000 paid to private insurers is a form of tax. To put it another way, Americans spend an average of $12,914 per person for healthcare compared with the European peer average of $6,125 per person. Since 60% of healthcare costs come from taxes, Americans already pay more in taxes for healthcare–$7,748—than do European peers. Moreover, the current combination of private premiums and FICA taxes is highly regressive. For instance, a secretary making $50,000 a year pays the same $6,000 premium as does someone working for the same employer who makes $125,000 per year. Experts estimate that universal healthcare, supported by some form of progressive taxes, will cost the middle class a little less and the wealthy a little more.

That Americans value choice is another reason given against universal healthcare; however, about 75% of Americans are enrolled in managed care plans that restrict individual choice to hospitals, physicians and other in-network services. With employers changing insurers almost annually, very few patients are able to keep long-term relationships with their providers. The final "against" reason is the assumption universal healthcare is an entitlement and the people who don't have health insurance are "deadbeats." Behind this assumption is the belief that healthcare is a commodity, like a truck or a toaster, not a social good, and therefore, those who use healthcare should pay for it. However, behind this belief lies another belief, "I've got mine and I don't want to pay for you."

Finally, free marketeers claim that the free market can control healthcare costs. There are several reasons why this has never worked and will never work. First, costs cannot be control when the motive is to profit quarterly. Because of the design of the U.S. healthcare system, any cost savings in one part is not used to reduce total healthcare costs but becomes the profits for that part. Moreover, the free-market cannot unite the parts of a fragmented healthcare system. Only a global budget can unite the U.S. system's fragmented parts into one, universal system. As other wealthy countries have consistently demonstrated, a non-profit, universal healthcare system gives everyone access to healthcare at an affordable price, where patients can choose their own providers, and providers are paid the same for the same services.

## Questions for the Reader

The questions provide an opportunity to examine your own mental models and values and to imagine other stakeholders' beliefs, fears, and values.

1 Does healthcare costs too much? Why do you believe this: what might others believe?
2 How much have your insurance premiums and out-of-pocket costs increased in the past five years?
3 If you have health insurance, should you have to worry about the affordability of out-of-pocket costs? Do you think you should know exactly what benefits your insurance covers and your out-of-pocket costs so that you can shop for the care at a price you can afford? Why; what might others believe?
4 If you are worried that you can't afford the care, can you talk with your doctor about the cost of your care? Can you speak up if there's a medicine you can't afford or a test your insurance won't cover? If yes, what were the results? If no, why can't you talk with your doctor about the affordability of care?

5 Does your health insurance cover the kinds of care you need, such as special drugs or certain specialists, hearing and dental? If not, how does that make you feel?
6 Have you, or someone you know, had to change doctors because your doctor was no longer in your insurer's network, received a surprise bill, or had your insurer deny care? Do you want your insurance company to choose your doctors or tell your doctors how to practice medicine?
7 Have you, or someone you know, have trouble paying a medical bill, been denied care because of an unpaid medical bill, or declared bankruptcy due to medical expenses? If yes, what effect did this have on you and your family?
8 Have you ever participated in crowd-funding for someone in your community who needs help paying their medical bill? How did this make you feel?
9 Has your hospital dropped any services in the past few years or closed? What impact did this have on your community?
10 From your perspective, where is the waste in the U.S. healthcare system? Would other stakeholders agree with you?
11 From your perspective, why does healthcare cost more in America compared to peer countries?
12 If you had a magic wand, how would you redesign the U.S. healthcare system to make it more efficient and include everyone? Where would the money come from? Why might other stakeholders agree with your redesign?

## Notes

1 Wagner, E., McGough, M., Rakshit, S., Krutika, A., & Cox, C. (2024, January 23). How does health care spending in the US compare to other countries? *Peterson-KFF Health Systems Tracker*. https://www.healthsystemtracker.org/chart-collection/health-spending.
2 The State of the U.S. Health Insurance in 2022. (2022, September 29). The Commonwealth Fund. https://commonwealthfund.org/pubications.
3 Grogan, C.M. (2023). *Grow and Hide: The History of America's Health Care State.* New York: Oxford University Press. p. 3.
4 Grogan, C.M. (2023). *Grow and Hide: The History of America's Health Care State.* New York: Oxford University Press. p. 3.
5 A Data Book: Health Care Spending and the Medicare Program. (2023, July). *MedPac Data Book.* www.medpac.gov/document-type/data.
6 The Nation's Health Dollar ($4.3 Trillion), Calendar Year 2021: Where It Went, Where It Came…, (2021) *Centers for Medicare and Medicaid Services.* https://www.cms.gov/files;documents/nations-health-dollar-where-it-came-from-where-it-went.
7 Shankosky, N., McDermott, D., & Kurani, N. (2020, August 12). How do US healthcare resources compare to other countries. *Peterson-KFF Health System Tracker*. www.healthsystemtracker.org/chart-collection/u-s-health-care-resources.
8 Peter G. Peterson Foundation. (2023, July 12). How does the U.S. health care system compare to other countries? https://www.pgpf.org/blog/2023/07/how.
9 Shrank, W.H., Rogstad, T.L., & Parekh, N. (2019, October 15). Waste in the US Health Care System: Estimated Costs and Potential for Savings. *JAMA Network.* https://jamanetwork.com/journals/jama/article-abstract/2752664.
10 Almost 25% of health care spending is considered wasteful. Here's why. (2023, April 3). https://www.pgpf.org/blog/2023/04/almost-.

11 Lopez, E., Neuman, T., Jacobson, G., & Levitt, L. (2020, April 15). How Much More Than Medicare Do Private Insurers Pay? A Review of the Literature. *Kaiser Family Foundation*. https://www.kff.org/medicare/issue-brief/how-much.
12 Uppal, N., Woolhandler, S., & Himmelstein, D.U. (2023, September 7). Alleviating medical debt in the United States. *New England Journal of Medicine*. 389 (10) 871–873.
13 Employer Health Benefits Survey, Section 1: Cost of Health Insurance-10020/KF. (2022, October 27). https://www.kff.org/report-section/ehbs-2022.
14 Statistica Research Department. (2023, December 18). Out-of-pocket health care spending in the U.S. – statistics and facts. https://www.statistica.com/topics/8223/out-of-pocket.
15 Unrelenting Pressure Pushes Rural Safety Net into Uncharted Territory. (2024, February). *The Chartis Group*. https://www.chartis.com/sites/default/files.
16 Dydra, L. (2024, February 16). 382 rural hospitals cut chemotherapy, breakdown by state. *Beckers Hospital Review*. https://www.beckershospitalreview.com/rankings-and.
17 Becker's Clinical Leadership & Infection Control. (2023, January 31). 45% of women forego preventive care: 7 notes. https://www.beckershospitalreview.com/patient.
18 Emerson, J. (2024, March 7). Large health system vs payer profits in 2023. https://www.beckershospitalreview.com/finance.
19 Emerson, J. (2024, March 7). Large health system vs payer profits in 2023. https://www.beckershospitalreview.com/finance.
20 Muoio, D. (2024, February 26). Despite sector-wide financial recovery, not all hospitals are finding their footing. *Fierce Healthcare*. https://www.fiercehealthcare.com/providers/despite.

# 3 Fifty Years of Cost Reductions Increased Costs

## A Very Brief History of Health Insurance

Health insurance as we know it in the U.S. emerged during the Great Depression. Before then, healthcare was mostly supplied by solo practitioners charging whatever the market would bear, the wealthy paid more, and the less wealthy paid less, and the poor—if they received care—received either public or charity care. Typically, hospitals were either public or private: public, or tax supported, for the indigent; voluntary, or private—usually sponsored by a religious organization—for those who could pay the generally affordable price.

However, the economic contraction of the Great Depression was a game changer. Many, who could previously afford healthcare, could no longer afford it. As a result, people either went without healthcare, or they weren't able to pay for it, or they had to pay on time. To stabilize their finances, Baylor Hospital in Dallas, Texas offered school teachers twenty-one days of hospital care for the prepayment of $6 per month. Because the plan gave Baylor a guaranteed revenue stream, other hospitals quickly followed suit, as did some employers. Overcoming their long-standing resistance to any form of health insurance, the American Medical Association (AMA), in 1942, finally approved of health insurance for *medical* care. By 1950, slightly more than half of the working public had some form of health insurance that covered hospital and medical care.

## Medicare Opens the Floodgates and Business Pushes Back

In the 1950s, U.S. healthcare costs were similar to those of other wealthy countries. Following the 1965 enactment of Medicare with its generous cost-plus, fee-for-service reimbursement, U.S. healthcare costs began to rise. Adding fuel to the fire, Medicare also accelerated the rise in costs by paying for-profit hospitals more than non-profits, stimulating the entry of for-profit hospitals into the market.

By 1973, large businesses were no longer willing to absorb the costs of healthcare into their production costs. General Motors famously claimed they spent more on healthcare than on steel for their vehicles. In the early 1970s, business was facing the lowest level of corporate profits since World War II, but healthcare—due to the nascent influx of Medicare money—was booming. Sympathetic to businesses'

DOI: 10.4324/9781003538226-4

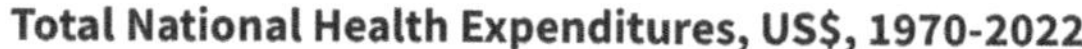


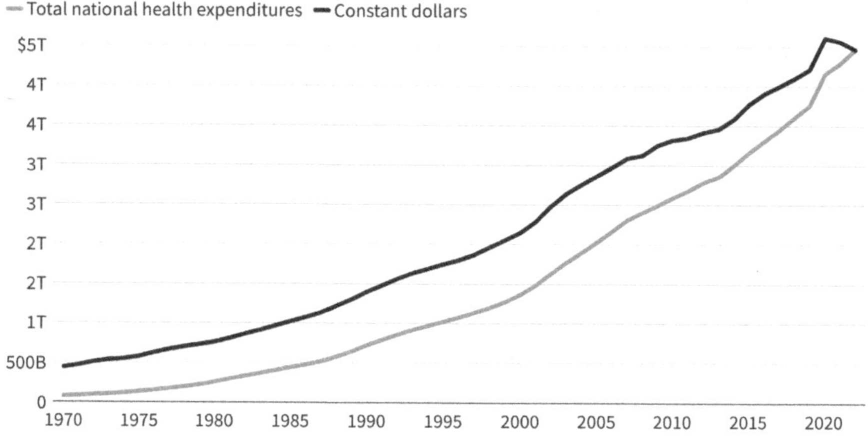


*Figure 3.1* Total National Health Expenditures, 1970–2022[1]

interests and, as the largest purchaser of healthcare, the federal government was also interested in reducing its healthcare costs. Along with widespread concerns over costs and inefficiencies, there were also growing concerns about uneven access to care and criticisms about poor health outcomes.

During the Nixon administration, there was talk of national health insurance, but policy analysts proposed that costs could be controlled by making healthcare responsive to market forces. Under the banner of "make healthcare function like a business," fifty years of piecemeal economic reforms have been tried and have failed, ultimately making healthcare more expensive. From the Nixon administration forward, policy changes to hold down healthcare costs failed. Between 1970 and 2022 healthcare costs rose from $74.1 billion to $4.465 trillion dollars (Figure 3.1).

## In 1970, Healthcare Spending Was $74.1 Billion and Per Capita Cost Was $353[2]

In 1973, to control overall healthcare costs, the Nixon administration enacted the Health Maintenance Organization (HMO) legislation, which gave birth to managed care. The legislation pursued market mechanisms—investment incentives, deregulation, and competition. Briefly, HMOs and other forms of managed care control costs by creating networks of approved hospitals, doctors, and other medical services who accept discounted rates. At the heart of an HMO are the primary care providers—family practitioners, pediatricians, and internists—who manage healthcare spending by emphasizing preventive care and managing chronic conditions, and by serving as the "gate-keeper" for access to tests, surgery, prescription drugs, and specialty care. Patients, too, were incentivized to control costs through the use of co-pays to discourage excess use of services. In the early 1970s, federal investment capital simultaneously stimulated growth of HMOs and managed care; it also incentivized their privatization. For about a decade, HMOs did hold down their part of healthcare costs.

Throughout the 1970s, business was actively involved in the redesign of healthcare financing. Purchasing coalitions were developed, giving business the power of numbers. The coalitions that represented the greatest number of employees typically received the greatest discount from insurance carriers. The Employee Retirement Income Security Act (ERISA), for which big business lobbied, gave business the right to be self-insured or self-funded. Briefly, this means businesses use the money they would have paid to an insurer to cover their employees' healthcare claims, while usually hiring a health insurer to manage the benefits. Because the business is not part of a larger risk pool but is paying only for the healthcare costs of their own employees, self-funding gives businesses an opportunity to save money.

Since being self-funding took business away from healthcare insurers, insurers responded by lobbying for deregulation in the insurance industry. Deregulation opened the door to for-profit insurers, although it took twenty years for the last insurer to become a for-profit enterprise. Deregulation also allowed insurers to abandon their tradition of community ratings for risk-segregated ratings, where each tranche is expected to be profitable. With community ratings, risks are pooled and the costs are shared with the understanding that I may not need healthcare today, but I might tomorrow. In contrast, with risk-segregated ratings, premiums are not based on the cost of caring for people over their life span but are calculated, per tranche, by age, gender, likelihood of disease, geography, etc. With each risk tranche expected to make a profit, younger people and males pay less and older people and women pay more for health insurance.

## In 1980, Healthcare Spending Was $253 Billion and Per Capita Cost Was $1,099[3]

In 1980, to control hospital costs, the Reagan administration replaced Medicare/Medicaid's cost-plus, fee-for service reimbursement with the prospective payment system (PPS), which commercial insurers quickly adopted. Fee-for-service reimbursement, which is the traditional model of payment, pays providers for *each* itemized service provided. By paying for volume, fee-for-service reimbursement implicitly incentivizes providers to provide more services because payment is based on the quantity not quality of care.

With PPS, instead of paying for *each* itemized service provided, payment is bundled and providers are paid a fixed amount, calculated according to a comprehensive formula. The PPS system is based on grouping medical diagnosis into related categories. Known as Diagnostic-Related Groups (DRGs), each group is assigned a pre-established payment for an episode of care. The payment is based on the medical severity of the DRG and the services typically used in its treatment. For instance, reimbursement for a heart attack, which typically uses more services, is greater than for a broken leg, which uses fewer services. Payment is further modified according to the patient's age and the presence of other health problems (comorbidities) secondary to the patient's medical problem.

In contrast to fee-for-service, PPS controls costs by incentivizing high quality, efficient care that avoids unnecessary tests and other services. In other words, the right care, at the right amount, at the right time. With PPS, providers make a profit by controlling their costs of caring for the patient. Generally, this means using fewer resources and discharging the patient earlier—patients are expected to recover at home once they were considered medically stable. Providers whose costs are less than the PPS payment make a profit. If the care costs more, the provider loses money. PPS doesn't always work as well in practice as in theory. For instance, sometimes patients feel they've been discharged too soon; sometimes patients are too sick to be discharged within the DRG schedule. Either way, providers are at risk.

With PPS, in-hospital care dropped as hospitals quickly pivoted from in-patient care to out-patient care that was still paid by fee-for-service. Ironically, the two different payment systems—one for in-patients and one for out-patients—coupled with investment incentives written into the Nixon and Reagan legislation opened a lucrative new market in out-patient care. Despite claims of patient convenience and lower costs, the burgeoning out-patient market of surgery, imaging, birthing, and urgent care centers duplicate existing hospital services and administrative overhead, further adding to expensive excess capacity and the overall cost of care.

Compounding the costly damage, investor owned out-patient facilities pull profitable services away from hospitals, leaving them with less operating capital to underwrite the needed, but poorly reimbursed services, such as emergency, intensive care, and obstetric services. To re-level the playing field, Congress, in 1997, authorized Centers for Medicare and Medicaid (CMS) to change the payment for out-patient care from fee-for-service to Outpatient Prospective Payment System (OPPS), which was implemented in 2000.

### In 1990, Healthcare Spending Was $718.8 Billion and Per Capita Cost Was $2,835[4]

When Clinton was elected, about 15% of working Americans didn't have health insurance. To make healthcare more affordable for everyone, the Clinton administration introduced The Health Act, in 1993. This enormous piece of legislation included insurance reform, universal coverage, and a basic, standardized slate of covered benefits that included mental health. Cost control was to be achieved through market reforms, which morphed into managed care. Responding to well-organized pushback from special interest groups—the AMA, the health insurance industry, political conservatives, and business—Congress said, "No," to Clinton's Health Act.

Despite the resounding "No" to The Health Act, the Clinton administration did get Congress to pass the Children Health Insurance Program (CHIP) legislation, a public plan that provides health insurance for children whose families earn too much to qualify for Medicaid but too little to afford private insurance. CHIP is a popular and needed program. In 1997, 15% of American children were uninsured.

In 2023, only 5% of American children were uninsured, and for children with insurance, 36% are insured either through CHIP or Medicaid.

Although Clinton's efforts for universal healthcare failed, cost-cutting legislation prevailed. One of the purposes of the Balanced Budget Act, passed by Congress in 1997, was to reduce Medicare and Medicaid costs. Among the reductions for hospitals were the implementation of OPPS payment for out-patient services and payment cuts for capital expenses. Equally significant, and for the first time, the CMS cut back its payments to physicians and hospitals. The Balanced Budget Act also expanded the states' discretion in administering Medicaid and the creation of Medicare+ Choice, a managed care version of Medicare privately purchased by seniors.

Because managed care gave insurers the ability to selectively contract with hospitals and physicians, insurers, for the first time, had more power than physicians. To gain more negotiating leverage, hospitals began employing physicians and independent hospitals began consolidating into large hospital systems, setting off the first wave of hospital mergers and acquisitions. Despite the putative cost cutting activities, healthcare's cost rose during the 1990s at double the rate of inflation. By the end of the 1990s, 44 million Americans, 16%, didn't have health insurance.

### In 2000, Healthcare Spending Was $1,365.7 Trillion and Per Capita Cost Was $4844[5]

In response to rising drug costs of the 1990s and because seniors complained that Medicare A and B didn't cover prescription drugs, the G.W. Bush administration enacted the Medicare Modernization Act. A significant updating of the Medicare program, the 2003 Act established prescription drug coverage, known as Medicare D, and replaced Medicare+ Choice with Medicare Advantage. Despite some members of Congress wanting to expand traditional Medicare to cover pharmaceutical drugs, the winners were the health insurance companies and pharmacy benefits managers who gained a larger role in Medicare's future.

For the first time, seniors had drug coverage through Medicare D. That's the good news. But there's plenty of bad news. First, Medicare D is a *private* plan that seniors had to purchase for themselves. Second, lobbying from the pharmaceutical and insurance industries prevented the federal government from negotiating the price of Medicare D or the price seniors would pay for their drugs.

For a few years, Medicare D made drugs more affordable for seniors. However, once pharmaceutical companies began to take advantage of the incentives built into the legislation, costs began to rise. Since the legislation prohibited Medicare from negotiating drug prices with pharmaceutical companies and since seniors were not paying full retail price but only their cost-sharing amounts, pharmaceutical companies felt free to significantly raise their prices. Insurers reacted by increasing the seniors' cost-sharing fees. As a result of this deliberate lack of systemic brakes, the average annual cost of brand name drugs rose threefold between 2006 and 2015, far exceeding the rate of inflation. As with all cost-shifting reactions, the costs are born by the patient, in this case, the senior. Between 2003 and 2024, millions of seniors struggled with prescription drug costs. In 2024, Congress enacted a spending cap, limiting Medicare beneficiaries' out-of-pocket expenses for prescription drugs to $2,000.

Although purported to control Medicare costs, Medicare Advantage has increased healthcare costs. Unlike traditional Medicare, which is a public plan, Medicare Advantage is a private, managed care insurance plan that includes pharmaceutical drug coverage and, depending on the price of the policy, may include other covered benefits, such as vision, dental, and gym memberships. It's funded by two revenue streams—public Medicare monies and private premiums plus out-of-pocket costs paid by seniors. Although its ads often claim very low premium costs, the *advantage* is to the insurance companies.

With Medicare Advantage premium costs, as well as co-pays, deductibles, and other forms of cost sharing are not standardized, but vary, depending on the senior's zip code and the benefits of the chosen plan. The trade-off for a lower plan premium usually includes higher cost-sharing and more restrictions on the use of services. Unlike traditional Medicare, Medicare Advantage doesn't travel. Except for emergency care, seniors are locked into narrow provider networks. Medicare Advantage, unlike traditional Medicare, is also fraught with denials and preauthorization requirements, a hassle for providers and patients alike.

Like the HMO legislation of 1970s, which incentivized private insurance, the Medicare Modernization Act did the same. As a result, private equity and venture capital continue to pour into Medicare Advantage plans. By 2023, slightly more than 50% of seniors use Medicare Advantage plans and the number is expected to rise. Its low premium fees make Medicare Advantage attractive to low income and People of Color. But, there's no free lunch. The adage "pay me now or pay me later, but you will pay" sums up the false economy of Medicare Advantage. The "pay me later" often comes *after* the hospitalization or out-patient care when the patient is surprised by the costliness of his cost-sharing portion of the medical bill. Unfortunately, the patient often pays thrice. First, he pays his share of the bill. Second, he pays with his health as the emotional and financial stress have an adverse effect on health and healing. Finally, he pays with his financial security. High out-of-pocket costs can deplete a patient's savings, damage his credit rating, and make it harder to pay his other bills.

Medicare Advantage plans are advertised as holding down the federal government's healthcare costs through narrow networks and preauthorizations; however, the actual results are not so clear. These plans have been heavily criticized. Berwick and Gilfillan have called them a "money machine," with a perverse business model that makes the plan overpaid and incorrectly paid—a model that costs the taxpayer dearly. Although the Medicare Modernization Act was touted to hold down Medicare costs, the major parts of the bill were written by lobbyists for insurance and drug companies, for their benefit. Their success is measured by Medicare expenses growing from $221.8 billion in 2000 to $522.9 billion in 2010.

Business also benefited from G.W. Bush's The Medicare Modernization Act. To reduce the amount of money employers spent on health insurance, The Act also included the language for "consumer-driven" health insurance. These are high-deductible plans coupled with a health savings account, which lets people use pre-tax dollars to help pay for medical expenses. The putative benefits were instead of paying higher premiums for insurance coverage people might not use, they (1) would shop for lower-priced insurance plans that met their medical needs, (2) shop for medical care, when needed, that offered the most affordable price, and (3) use money from the health savings account to pay for uncovered medical care.

The reality is patients don't have crystal balls. Who can forecast his future health needs? Shopping for gallbladder surgery is not like shopping for a new Ford. The hospital's prices, although supposedly transparent, are difficult to interpret. However, affordability also depends upon one's out-of-pocket costs after the insurance has paid its part, which usually comes as a surprise since most people assume they have "good" insurance. People seldom have the luxury of time to shop if the service is needed now; and choices are very limited in rural areas. Moreover, all medical care is out-of-pocket until the deductible is met. If the deductible is too high, people forego care, even urgently needed healthcare. Between 2007 and 2020, the percent of workers having a high-deductible plan has grown from 4% to 53%. While these plans have lowered employers' healthcare costs, they have left many Americans underinsured and afraid to access necessary healthcare.

## In 2010, Healthcare Spending Was $2,589.4 Trillion and the Per Capita Cost Was $8380[6]

In 2010 about 16% of Americans didn't have health insurance, representing a thirty-year high of uninsured working Americans. In 2010, the Patient Protection Affordable Care Act was enacted by the Obama administration.

Commonly known as "Obamacare" and abbreviated as the Affordable Care Act (ACA), the purpose of the plan was to make affordable health insurance available to more people and to "bend the cost curve." Originally, the plan required Americans to obtain health insurance. This was to be accomplished by (1) requiring businesses with fifty or more employees to provide health insurance, (2) creating health insurance exchanges, and (3) encouraging states to expand Medicaid. The plan also included reforming the insurance industry, and supporting innovative care delivery models and reimbursement schemes to reduce overall healthcare costs.

Some of the popular benefits of the ACA include allowing children younger than twenty-six to stay on their parent's health plan; no co-pays for some kinds of preventive services; and the elimination of annual and lifetime caps on healthcare spending, which prohibit insurers from limiting yearly or lifetime coverage for medical expenses. For instance, many patients hospitalized in ICUs with COVID-19 had hospital bills of over $1 million, a common lifetime cap prior to the ACA. Had the cap not been eliminated, the patient would have been responsible for the amount over $1 million and, most likely, uninsurable the rest of his life.

To expand affordable health insurance, the ACA created health exchanges, which are owned and operated by private insurers. Federal subsidies are available to help low-income people purchase private insurance from the health exchange. The ACA also encouraged states to expand Medicaid to cover those whose income was too high to qualify for Medicaid but too low to buy from the health exchange. States were incentivized to expand Medicaid by shifting the Medicaid reimbursement from, essentially, a 50/50 state/federal responsibility to 10% state and 90% federal responsibility. The ACA required insurers to cover ten essential benefits and make preventive care a covered benefit. It also required insurers to spend at least 85% of their premium funds on medical coverage. This was a significant change since insurers previously spent about 65% of premium funds on medical coverage with the remaining 35% spent on CEO salaries, marketing, and investor dividends.

Despite the intensive opposition and the shibboleths declaiming the ACA was "socialized medicine," the ACA legislation was basically written by the insurance industry for the insurance industry. Although the law is not perfect and it did not control costs, the number of uninsured dropped by 10 million in its first year.

## In 2016, Healthcare Spending Was $3,307.4 Trillion and Per Capita Cost Was $10,247[7]

During the Trump administration the number of uninsured rose by about a million people per year. Congress made numerous failed attempts to "repeal and replace Obamacare" with something "cheaper and better." During that time, however, many small changes were made to the ACA. Some of these small changes included removing penalties for not buying health insurance; allowing states to add work requirements to Medicaid; incentivizing seniors to purchase Medicare Advantage by reducing premium costs; and introducing minimum essential coverage (MEC) plans, or "skinny" plans.

MEC plans are attractive because of their low premiums. However, as the names—minimum and skinny—suggest, MEC plans are a far cry from traditional health insurance. MEC plans generally cover wellness and preventive tests, low-cost care. However, these bare-bone plans do not cover out-patient care or hospitalizations. Sadly, it's after a serious illness or hospitalization people discover their plan left them financially exposed, a painful stress no one needs when recovering from a serious illness.

## In 2020, Healthcare Spending Was $4,124 Trillion and Per Capita Cost Was $12,530[8]

Compared with 2019, the year 2020 registered a noticeable jump in costs compared to the national spending of $3,701 trillion and a per person cost of $11,462. Throughout the 2010s, healthcare spending grew about 4% annually. When COVID-19 hit, healthcare spending jumped 9.7% between 2019 and 2020, due to the federal government's response to the pandemic. Generally speaking, increased federal spending included the Provider Relief Fund, which helped hospitals and other providers stay in business, and the Paycheck Protection program, which helped others stay in business. Extra funds were also spent on public health, which included COVID-19 testing and vaccine development, payment to hospitals for treating uninsured patients with COVID-19, and for increased Medicaid enrollment as laid-off workers became eligible for Medicaid.

In contrast to the increase in federal spending, in 2020, private insurance spending dropped and the public's out-of-pocket costs dropped slightly, owing to the public's lower use of regular healthcare services during the pandemic. Despite the increase in federal spending during 2020 and 2021, 40% of U.S. hospitals still had negative profit margins due to a combination of high labor, drug, and supply costs; reimbursements from Medicare and Medicare that don't cover the cost of care; and private insurers extensive use of preauthorization to deny and delay access to care.

For the remainder of the 2020s, CMS projects healthcare spending to increase about 5.4% annually. Although unfortunate and troublesome, the hangover from COVID-19 is still present. At the end of 2023, the effects of inflation and the Great Resignation made returning to "normal" more wishful thinking than probable. Other potentially expensive COVID-19-related factors include increased and unprecedented behavioral health needs; serious health disparities among the poor and People of Color; and the rapid entry of digital medicine.

Likewise, the ongoing vertical and horizontal consolidation of healthcare due to the flood of venture capital and private equity seeking high returns for their investments, the consolidation among hospitals, insurers, and physician specialty practices; and the entry of retail health, such as CVS and Amazon, are projected to accelerate this decade's healthcare costs.

Finally, health insurance costs are projected to rise in 2024, to almost $24,000 for a family policy. This is an 8.5% price hike, double the rate of 2023. Reasons include inflation, more people with more chronic and expensive conditions, and the availability of significantly more expensive drugs, such as Ozempic for weight loss and targeted therapy drugs for cancer treatment. While it's too early to tell how the Biden administration will address rising healthcare costs, the forecast is for more of the same: more government subsidizes and limited governmental attempts to control drug costs for seniors, and a few state and federal restrictions on insurance companies regarding surprise billing and prior authorization.

## The Corporatization of Healthcare

Starting in the 1970s, the combination of federal dollars from Medicare's Fee for service (FFS) reimbursement, healthcare's generous profit margins, and the loosening of federal regulations made healthcare attractive to investors. In less than two decades, investment incentives shifted healthcare away from solo practitioners and stand-alone, nonprofit hospitals and insurers to corporate conglomerates. This attractiveness opened the door to mergers and acquisitions as well as reinforced the growth of investor-owned national chains of for-profit hospitals, nursing homes, physician management companies, and out-patient services, to name a few. Not to be left out, community and non-profit hospitals also took advantage of the economies of scale, better negotiation leverage, better access to capital, better supply chain management, and the reduction of fiscal risk that come with corporatization. By 2022, of the 5,129 community hospitals, 24% are investor owned, 18%

are state or locally owned, and 58% are non-profit, of which 68% are part of a large hospital system.[9]

Corporatization profoundly increased hospitals' and physicians' administrative burden. Managing the business of healthcare requires additional layers of bureaucracy and costly technology, as well as more overseers and more sophisticated administrators. Corporatization also generated legions of record-keeping personnel and new industries of consultants, increasing the number of healthcare employees as lawyers, accountants, lobbyists, human resources experts, marketing specialists, software programmers, and so forth needed to manage the business of healthcare. Between 1970 and 1991, the number of healthcare administrators in the U.S. increased by 697%, compared to a 129% increase in clinical personnel.[10] The number keeps growing. Between 2001 and 2016, over 4 million net new jobs were added,[11] resulting in twice the number of administrative staff as there are doctors and nurses. In comparison, other American service industries, such as education and legal, typically have about 0.85 administrative workers for each professional employee.[12]

Although corporatization promised cost control and increased efficiency, that hasn't been the outcome. Instead, the consolidation within the healthcare industry—insurers, large hospital systems, and employed physician groups—has resulted in what some consider monopolies and a concomitant result in less competition along with higher prices. Today, non-profit insurance companies are a thing of the past and about 75% of physicians are employed. The business practices of for-profit and non-profit hospitals are fundamentally similar. Their primary difference—non-profits don't pay taxes and for-profits pay stockholder dividends. The similarity of business practices has also reached the board room. According to Jamie Orlikoff writing for an AHA magazine for hospital boards, between 2018 and 2022, the number of non-profit and for-profit hospitals that compensated their boards doubled, from 13% to 27%. In contrast, by 2022, 34% of large systems' boards were compensated, a huge increase from the 3% who compensated their boards in 2018.[13]

### Market Failure

Under the banner of "make healthcare function like a business," fifty years of market corrections—deregulation, new IRS rules, prioritization of shareholder value, easy access to investment capital, and new financial tools—have had a perverse effect. Healthcare's costs increased sixfold.

A purely competitive market is characterized by three ideals: ideal competition, ideal information, and ideal price. Ideal competition assumes a market place with a large number of competing producers and free, or unrestricted, entry for new producers. Ideal information assumes that consumers have complete information about the price and quality of the product. Lastly, ideal price assumes there is one optimal price—the balance of production costs and price—adjusted in accordance with supply and demand.

Healthcare inherently violates all three ideals. On the supply side, entry isn't free. One can't simply open a hospital or say "I'm a doctor." On the demand side, patients don't have complete information about price and quality. Employers, not the patient, typically purchase health insurance, not the patient. Thus, the employer controls his costs by passing more of the cost to the employee through high deductibles, coinsurance, and co-pays, costs that generally change annually depending upon the vagaries of the market place. And, physicians, not the patient, determine how much and what kind of care is purchased. In commodity markets, the consumer can determine whether he needs a new truck and how much he's willing to pay. Unlike buying a new truck, however, patients don't plan for cancer or a broken leg, or any other malady. For the most part, they cannot forecast their healthcare needs. Nor can patients wait for sales, nor can they say, "I'll take the used truck version of the gallbladder surgery because I can't afford the new one." The reason people have insurance is to cover those unexpected costs.

On the supply side, the most efficient way to make money in a free market is to reduce production costs. But, in a fragmented healthcare system, reducing production costs means avoiding the sick and poor people, denying, delaying and limiting care, and closing costly services—behaviors contradictory to the purpose of healthcare. These cost controlling behaviors are considered moral injuries by physicians and contribute to physician burnout. In a purely competitive market, competition disciplines *all* players equally. Because of the fragmented structure of the U.S. healthcare system, all players cannot be disciplined equally. As a result, the largest players—such as insurance and pharmaceutical conglomerates, and large hospital systems—prosper while the most in need of services—patients—are the most vulnerable to exclusion and have the highest out-of-pocket costs.

## Fifty Years of Cost-Cutting Redux

As fifty years of "cost-controlling" legislation have demonstrated, free market principles cannot control healthcare costs (Figure 3.2). Between 1970 and 2020, healthcare costs rose from $74.1 billion to $4.5 trillion, a sixty-fold increase, representing 6.9% of the GDP in 1970 and 19.5% in 2020. Using 2019 data, 60% of healthcare expenditures are paid for by public funds.[14]

The piecemeal healthcare legislation and regulation are rational and essentially do what they were intended to do: optimize a particular part of the healthcare system. However, as fifty years of rising costs demonstrate, the optimization of a part comes at the expense of the whole. Because the U.S. healthcare system is for-profit and a highly fragmented system, fifty years of "cost cutting" legislation have served the self-interest of various special interest groups.

Unfortunately, the lack of concern about the whole, coupled with the lack of systemic controls to equitably hold down costs throughout the entire system, maintains our fragmented healthcare system. Fragmentation reinforces winners and losers. Fragmentation also reinforces an economic relationship between self-interest groups and politicians where there's a pay-off. Those who contribute the most toward politicians' elections receive the power of the state to achieve their own self-interest. These results are inescapable in a for-profit system. Over a fifty-year period, healthcare's traditional altruistic values have given way to financial values.

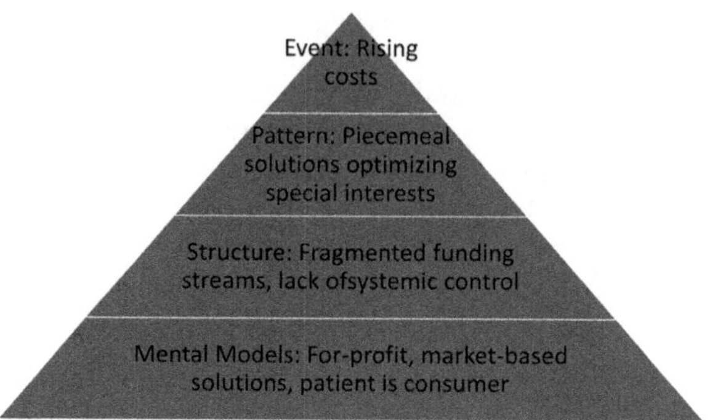


*Figure 3.2* Iceberg Model: Market Failure

Americans would have been better served had the policy analysts taken a systemic approach. Had they done so they would have seen that costs can't be controlled in a fragmented system with multiple funding streams and its major stakeholders—hospitals, physicians, pharmaceutical companies, and insurers—competing with each other and among themselves. This fragmented, competitive structure results in cost shifting, duplication of services, and duplication of administrative overhead, which add to the U.S.'s higher costs. The brunt of these costs is borne by the public who consistently pay more for healthcare through higher premiums and out-of-pocket costs, and through their taxes.

## How Other Wealthy Countries Control Healthcare Costs

Other wealthy, capitalist countries control healthcare costs in four ways. First, their organizing mental model is healthcare is a social good, not a commodity, or to put it another way, healthcare is a right, not a privilege. Second, peer countries have non-profit healthcare systems. Third, they have an integrated structure: the various stakeholders—insurers, patients, providers, and the pharmaceutical industry—are parts in the *same* system. Concomitantly, peer countries have universal healthcare so everyone has access to healthcare. Fourth, they balance the relationships among the system's parts: They all use a global budget to control costs and discipline all players equally. While no system is perfect, all, but Great Britain and Switzerland, have a mix of public and private funded, governmental regulated healthcare systems, which have much better health outcomes at about half the cost of the U.S. healthcare system.

For decades, the cries of "socialized medicine" and "don't trust the government" have been used to defeat any kind of universal healthcare in the U.S. Yet, veterans generally like the healthcare provided by the Veterans Administration and seniors generally like traditional, or Medicare A and B. VA medical care is socialized medicine in that the government owns the buildings, employs the physicians and other clinicians, and pays for care using taxpayer money. Similarly, traditional Medicare, which is like the Canadian healthcare system, is single-payer system where the government uses public tax money to pay private providers; and its overhead costs are much less than private insurance.

## Questions for the Reader

The questions provide an opportunity to examine your own mental models and values and to imagine other stakeholders' beliefs, fears, and values.

1. Should the U.S. healthcare system remain a for-profit system? What are the benefits, if any, of our for-profit system? Who are the winners and the losers with a for-profit healthcare system?
2. Should only people who can afford their healthcare bills have access to healthcare? Why do you believe this; what might others believe?
3. Should the uninsured and those who can't afford the out-of-pocket costs have access to healthcare? If yes, where should the money come from? Why; what might others believe?
4. Should the cost of insurance vary by age, gender, geography, and the employer's generosity? Why; what might others believe?
5. Most insurance pays for 80% of the bill, leaving the patient with the remaining 20%. The average ICU cost is about $10,000 per day; the average cost of treating breast cancer ranges from $20,000 to $100,00. Could you easily afford your 20%? Do you believe most people could? Is it fair that most insurance doesn't cover the full cost of care?
6. Who should determine what benefits are covered (what your insurance will pay for), your employer, your insurance company, the courts, religious organizations, state legislatures, federal government? Why?
7. From your perspective, why did fifty years of federal legislation designed to control healthcare costs not only fail but increased the number of systemic fractures? Why; what might others believe?
8. From your perspective, what are the downsides of not having one standardized form of insurance that reimburses all providers the same for the same procedure?
9. Should *all* employers be required to provide health insurance? Should employers cover the full premium costs? Should premiums cover the full cost of care? Why do you believe what you believe? Should the government subsidize your health insurance? Should it subsidize everyone's? Why; what might others believe?
10. Other wealthy countries essentially have one payment system and use a global budget to control costs, which their governments regulate. What are the upsides for the U.S. having one payment system and a global budget? What are the downsides?

## Notes

1 McGough, M., Winger, A., Rakshit, S., & Amin, K. (2023, December, 15). How has U.S. spending on healthcare changed over time? *Peterson-KFF Tracker*. https://www.healthsystemtracker.org/chart/collection/u-s-spending.

2 Amadeo, K. (2022, October 21). The rising cost of health care by year and its causes. T*he Balance*. https://www. thebalancemoney.com/causes-of-rising-healthcare-costs-4064878.
3 Amadeo, K. (2022, October 21). The rising cost of health care by year and its causes. T*he Balance*. https://www. thebalancemoney.com/causes-of-rising-healthcare-costs-4064878.
4 Amadeo, K. (2022, October 21). The rising cost of health care by year and its causes. T*he Balance*. https://www. thebalancemoney.com/causes-of-rising-healthcare-costs-4064878.
5 Amadeo, K. (2022, October 21). The rising cost of health care by year and its causes. T*he Balance*. https://www. thebalancemoney.com/causes-of-rising-healthcare-costs-4064878.
6 Amadeo, K. (2022, October 21). The rising cost of health care by year and its causes. T*he Balance*. https://www. thebalancemoney.com/causes-of-rising-healthcare-costs-4064878
7 Amadeo, K. (2022, October 21). The rising cost of health care by year and its causes. T*he Balance*. https://www. thebalancemoney.com/causes-of-rising-healthcare-costs-4064878.
8 Amadeo, K. (2022, October 21). The rising cost of health care by year and its causes. T*he Balance*. https://www. thebalancemoney.com/causes-of-rising-healthcare-costs-4064878
9 Fast Facts on U.S. Hospitals Infographics. (2024, January 12). *AHA*. https://www.aha.org/system/files/media/file/2024/.
10 Clanham-Clyne, J., Himmelstein, D., & Woolhandler, S. (1995). *The Regional Option for a National Health Program.* Stone Creek, CT: Pamphleteer's Press. p. 43.
11 Sahni, N.R., Kumar, P., Levine, E., & Singhal, S. (2019, February 27). The productive imperative for healthcare delivery in the United States. *McKinsey & Company.* https://www.mckinsey.com/industries/healthcare-systems-and-services/our-insights/the-productivity-imperative-for-healthcare-delivery-.
12 Sahni, N., Carrus, B., & Cutler, D.M. (2021, October 20). Administrative simplification and the potential for saving a quarter of a trillion dollars in health care. *JAMA Network.* https://www.jamanetwork.com/journals/fullarticle/2785480.
13 Orlikoff, J. (2023, December). Trustee Insights. Board compensation: The emerging new normal. *AHA Trustee Insights.* https://trustees.aha.org/board-compensation-emerging-new-normal.
14 Grogan, C.M. (2023). *Grow and Hide: The History of America's Health Care State.* New York: Oxford University Press. p. 3.

# 4 Creative Disruptors

## Creative Disruption

Popularized by the tech industry, creative disruption is an economic term attributed to the Austrian economist, Joseph Schumpeter. The term refers to radical changes in the market place brought about by innovation, taking a complex, high-priced product and replacing it with something more convenient and less expensive. For a long time, healthcare was immune to disruption. Just as a triangle is the strongest shape, the historical configuration of healthcare was triangle-like. Leaning on each other, doctors, hospitals, and insurers gave a three-sided strength to healthcare. Medical care was provided in-person by licensed physicians, whose licensing laws gave them monopoly power. Hospitals, known as the "doctors' workshops," provided the expensive technology. And, health insurance provided access and paid the bills.

As the financing of healthcare shifted, self-protecting moves by all three players have gradually weakened their iron triangle. For instance, better payment for out-patient care incentivized the growth of for-profit ambulatory surgery centers, imaging, birthing and infusion centers, and other freestanding services, taking profitable, low over-head services away from legacy hospitals and contributing to expensive duplication of services. Through consolidation and offering their own health plans, some large hospital systems have increased their bargaining power and competed with insurers, respectively. Finally, physicians, too, have engaged in self-protection. Responding to the increasing pressures of cost, complexity, and risk of being in private practice, physicians are seeking employment in hospitals and corporate practices. As of 2023, 77% of physicians were employed.[1]

## Nurse Practitioners

Sometimes known as mid-level practitioners, non-physician providers (NPPs) are healthcare professionals who are not physicians but have their own scope of practice. Depending on the laws of the state, NPPs either practice either independently, in collaboration with a physician, or under the supervision of a physician. Examples include physician assistants, nurse practitioners (NPs), certified nurse midwives, and certified registered nurse anesthetists.

DOI: 10.4324/9781003538226-5

Of the NPPs, NPs were an early disruptor of the physicians' monopoly over the delivery of care. With their own scope of practice and licensing laws, which vary by state, NPs can work independently from physicians in twenty-seven states. Although nurse practitioner training is different from physician training—a two-year master's degree compared to a four-year medical school degree and subsequent residency—NPs are licensed to diagnose and treat patients, order and interpret diagnostic tests and prescribe medications, and can directly bill insurance companies, depending on the requirements of the state and the insurer.

NPs entered the healthcare landscape about 1965, as a response to rural shortages and the uneven distribution of physicians. Their number begin rising in the 1990s, with the growth of managed-care and its use of NPs for cost containment. Since then, the number of NPs has grown steadily. Today, the U.S. has about 355,000 NPs, compared to a little over one million licensed physicians. Since the U.S. is now graduating more NPs per year than physicians, and since NPs take less training and are paid significantly less than physicians, NPs are expected to compensate for the growing doctor shortage—especially for primary care physicians.

Like physicians, NPs are licensed by the state in which they live. Based on their training, NPs can make diagnosis, order tests, manage treatment, and prescribe medications. Twenty-seven states allow NPs to practice independent of physician supervision. Nine states require NPs to work under a physician's supervision, and the remaining states have limited some aspect of the practitioner's independence.

By 2024, NPs are moving into specialty care where the pay is better than in primary care. Evidence shows the hoped for coverage of rural medicine hasn't worked because NPs have gravitated to the same desirable locations as physicians, leaving rural areas underserved. While NPs are here to stay, their acceptance is mixed. Proponents say NPs serve a vital role. They are often the only provider in rural and underserved urban communities. NPs can be important players in medical practices, when well-integrated. By seeing the less complex patients, NPs increase the patients' access to care, while adding value to the physician's practice.

However, there are few studies regarding their contribution and results are mixed.[2] For example, a veterans administration (VA) study shows the cost of diabetic care by nurse practitioners (NPs) and physician assistants (PAs) was 6% to 7% lower than provided by physicians whose patients had more hospitalizations and emergency department visits.[3] In contrast, data from an Accountable Care Organization in Hattiesburg, Mississippi showed the cost of care by NPs was higher than care provided by physicians. The more expensive NP care was attributed to more tests, more referrals to specialists, and more emergency department visits.[4]

Like most everything in healthcare, politics is in the mix. While nurses like the advance-practice autonomy and many see NPs as a solution to the physician shortage, especially in rural areas, the American Medical Association (AMA) is advocating for "physician-lead care." Adamantly against "scope-of-practice-expansions," the AMA strongly believes NPs should not function independently.[5] That said, if NPs become the low-cost providers for underserved areas, then the result is more fragmentation and a two-tiered system.

**Telehealth**

To be disruptive, technology must be easily available to the majority of its users and offer new and superior benefits. Although available prior to COVID-19, telehealth had been minimally used due to onerous regulatory and reimbursement rules. Once COVID-19 created the urgent need for patients to access care without the risk of being infected or infecting others, state and federal agencies quickly established emergency procedures that protected patients and physicians alike. Patients gained access to safe care and physicians got paid. With insurers required to pay physicians the same for telehealth visits as in-person care, many practices stayed solvent because of these emergency procedures.

Telehealth's convenience and accessibility (shorter wait times) are the disruptors. With telemedicine, patients can use their smart phone, iPad, or desktop to "see" their own physicians, or even a specialist in another state. This is done without the inconvenience of driving somewhere, waiting for the doctor to see them, and taking time off from work. Telemedicine also makes it easy for patients who do not have their own physician to shop online, using one of the direct-to-consumers telehealth companies for an easily accessible appointment and to avoid the long wait time and hassle of finding a local physician who is in their network and is taking new patients.

As COVID-19 drove up the incidence of depression and anxiety in adults and teens, telehealth has emerged as an ideal way to deliver behavioral health. It's convenient; it's private; appointments are available outside normal business hours; and it gives access to behavioral health services to the home-bound and those living in underserved areas. Besides the ease and convenience of "telepsych," its outcomes are equal to in-person care in terms of effectiveness and overall quality of care.[6]

Insurers are using telehealth to control costs. Many insurers are requesting patients use the insurer's online physicians, before seeing their more costly primary care physician or going to the even more costly emergency department. This cost savings for insurers are also less expensive and more convenient for patients. It's great for parents who are worried about a sick child in the middle of the night or are unable to take time off work for an office visit. Telehealth provides the convenience and access consumers have come to expect in other areas of their lives.

Despite its convenience and accessibility, telehealth isn't a panacea. Older adults, the poor, People of Color, and those living in rural areas may not have the needed technology. Health outcomes may not be as good for patients with multiple complex problems, or in cases requiring in-person examinations, such as listening to the patient's heart or when the patient can't report his vital signs because he doesn't have a thermometer or blood pressure cuff. Also, visual assessment may not be as good, such as examining a laceration to determine if stitches are needed.

COVID-19 catalyzed the rapid adoption of telehealth. Telemedicine is here to stay; however, the retiring federal, state, and emergency waivers raise three important questions about the best path forward. First, medical care has, historically, been delivered in-person at a defined bricks and mortar location; however, with telehealth care can be delivered from *anywhere*. This calls into question whether state licensing laws that protect physicians from out-of-state competition are out of date. Second, because telehealth's convenience and accessibility hold the potential for over-utilization of care, the question is how to encourage high-value care. High-value care is a term that refers care that optimizes a good outcome for the patient, but discourages over-utilization of care, which benefits the provider at the insurer's expense. The final question is about optimal reimbursement policies for going forward. For instance, should reimbursement be limited to certain services for selected patient populations and health conditions? Should reimbursement be on par with in-person visits? Should a doctor stationed in Ohio but "seeing" a patient in Wyoming be required to be licensed in Wyoming? Should telephone visits be reimbursed on par with video visits, especially since rural areas have better telephone than internet services? Although these questions are yet to be answered, insurers and providers are beginning to see that the convenience of telemedicine is something patients have come to expect.

## Healthcare Apps

Fueled by advances in technology, capital investments, and the ubiquity of smart phones, health apps are a growing trend. At least 20% of smart phone users have one or more health applications on their phones to track fitness, increase their wellness, access healthcare data, create medication reminders, access telehealth, review their medical records, monitor certain conditions remotely, and manage a specific medical condition. Since 2016 the U.S. digital market has steadily grown and is forecast to reach $50.17 billion in 2024.[7]

Varying from smart watches to dedicated devises, fitness trackers are wrist-worn technology that collects and measures data about the wearer's physical activity and health. Fitness trackers typically track physical activity, calories burned, hours slept, heart rate, blood pressure, and stress and mood. A large variety of self-help apps, at different prices and with different features, include smoking cessation, addiction recovery, weight loss, stress management, and pregnancy care, to name a few. Remote monitoring, however, lets providers monitor and manage a patient's blood pressure, heart rate, weight, oxygen levels, and other bio-data outside the traditional setting. While remote monitoring spares the patient the inconvenience of travel, these monitoring devises have built-in alerts that notify the patient's provider if the data falls outside the desired range, which enables providers to promptly adjust the patient's treatment before a problem turn into a crisis.

Finally, the most recent addition to the health app catalogue are the digital therapeutic apps. These unique apps are different in that they are evidence-based, therapeutic interventions for the prevention, management, and treatment of health conditions. Food and Drug Administration (FDA) approved and generally require a prescription, the devices are readily scalable and are suitable for a variety of indications, such as diabetes, respiratory diseases, pain management, and mental health that require traditional pharmaceutic management as well as engaged self-care. For instance, an app connects a smart phone to a continuous glucose monitor (CGM). The CGM, which replaces glucose meters, test strips, etc., is a disc about the size of a nickel and sticks to the skin like a Band Aid and allows diabetics to monitor their blood glucose in real time. The app alarms if blood glucose levels are too high or too low. By displaying trends over time and allowing for notes about food and exercise, the real-time information enables patients to be more knowledgeable about and proactively engaged with the management of their chronic condition.

Health apps are disrupting the practice and reach of health care. Like all healthcare technology, health apps are big business with their own set of pros and cons. The pros include ease of use and convenience; improve the patient's understanding of his disease; improve patient engagement with his own care; allow providers to remotely monitor a patient's condition and the early detection of arising problems; and improve health outcomes. Remote monitoring and digital therapeutic apps have extended access to care beyond the traditional four walls and may bring care to more patients at a lower cost. Lastly, by improving self-care engagement and improved health outcomes, digital therapeutic apps may free up system capacity, alleviating provider shortages. The cons include data privacy risk; confusion due to too many choices; uneven insurance coverage and affordability, although some apps are free. Other problems stem from lack of experience. For example, regulatory oversight and approval are in their infancy, as is research regarding their effect on health outcomes and the integration of health apps into provider systems.

## Artificial Intelligence

Artificial intelligence (AI) is boldly claiming it will revolutionize healthcare. Several of its claims deserve special mention. One is its machine learning algorithms will lead to earlier detection of diseases, increased speed and accuracy of diagnosis, and precision treatment, or care that is customized to the patient's genetic background, medical history, and lifestyle. Another is to increase overall efficiencies, such as improving workflows and automating repetitive tasks. Because AI has the power to analyze vast quantities of data, AI has the potential to expedite pharmaceutical research and development, as well as the potential for early identification and tracking of infectious diseases and monitoring mitigation strategies efficiencies.

With AI still in its early stages of adoption, the degree to which AI can fulfill its transformative potential is still to be determined. Despite the optimism, AI is not without risks. Among the risks are its high costs, the technology is constantly evolving, and its current lack of interoperability. Other risks include possible security breaches, loss of patient privacy, and still to be answered questions about regulatory compliance, ethics, and who is legally liable when the use of AI causes patient harm.

## The Shkreli Effect

About 66% of adult Americans take one prescription drug daily, with about 25% taking four or more daily. Utilization is higher for older adults and those with chronic conditions. According to Centers for Medicare and Medicaid (CMS), U.S.

spending on prescription drugs has steadily increased, rising from $122 billion in 2000 to $358 billion in 2020.[8] This is an annual average per capita expense of about $1,126 compared to an annual average of $552 for eleven comparable countries.[9]

Although insurers pay the bulk of the average costs, there's no free lunch—high drug costs are passed on to the individual in the form of higher insurance premiums, higher co-pays, and deductibles. About 80% of Americans think that prescription drugs cost too much; 75% think drug companies' profits are too high; 30% have trouble affording the out-of-pocket costs; 16% don't fill a prescription because of costs; and 13% skipped doses or cut their medications in half to make the prescription last longer, according to a 2022 Kaiser Family Foundation survey.[10]

Prescription affordability is not an issue for people living in other wealthy countries, however. First, their citizens are protected from high out-of-pocket costs through their universal healthcare. Second, other wealthy countries control the prices pharmaceutical companies can charge. Although the specific methodology varies, these countries use a mix of regulatory and market-based mechanisms, including centralized price negotiations, national formularies, and regulated markups throughout the production and distribution supply chain. In the U.S., however, prices are set according to whatever the market will bear.

The infamous Martin Shkreli provides an egregious example of "whatever the market will bear." Overnight Shkreli, the CEO of Turing, a biopharmaceutical company that entered the market in 2015 raised the price of Daraprim from $13.50 to $750 per pill—a 5,000% jump in price. Daraprim is a generic drug that's been on the market a long time and is critical to the treatment of HIV. When Turing bought the rights to distribute the drug, it had been on the market a long time. Prior to 2010 it was priced at $1.00 per pill, rose to $13.50 when the distribution rights were sold the first time, and rose to $750 when the rights were sold to Turing.

When asked why, since the drug cost about a dollar to make, and had been priced at $13.50 for Shkreli's response was, "We need to turn a profit on this drug."[11] Although Shkreli was heavily criticized for price gouging, he went to jail for defrauding his investors. The point is, once Shkreli showed the prices older drugs that don't have generic rivals could be brought in line with newer, blockbuster drugs, other companies quickly followed suit, raising prices astronomically on drugs whose prices hadn't been raised in many years. For example, the EpiPen price increase, from $100 per two-pen pack to $600 over a ten-year period, caught the public's attention in 2016.

In 2024, private insurers and Medicare and Medicaid are struggling with how to pay for the highly expensive and highly popular, injectable weight loss drugs, Ozempic and Wegovy. They are two of the new, second generation, GLP-1 receptor agonists that are also used for the treatment of type two diabetes and may reduce the risk of stroke, heart disease, and other health problems associated with obesity. While hailed as miracle drugs, current studies indicate they must be taken forever or the weight will return. With the U.S. list price of over $1,200 per month and about forty percent of the U.S. population are obese, according to the Centers for Disease Control and Prevention (CDC), these popular drugs have the potential to drive up everyone's insurance costs and to bankrupt Medicare. As usual, Americans pay the most—ten times more than its peers. According to a report released by Bernie Sanders (I-Vt) of the Senate's Health, Labor, Education and Pension Committee, "there's no rational reason other than greed, for Novo Nordisk to charge Americans struggling with obesity $1,349 per month for Wegovy when this same exact product can be purchased for just $186 in Denmark, $137 in Germany, and $92 in the United Kingdom, which it costs less than $5 to profitably manufacture."[12]

The Shkreli effect represents the pharmaceutical industry's business model: Use taxpayer money for basic science research and development; prevent competition through patent protection laws; if one company raises its prices, raise yours as well; charge as much as the market will bear; discontinue low margin, generic drugs; enjoy very low tax rates due to loopholes in tax laws; increase economic leverage through market consolidation; increase political leverage through the use of lobbyists and campaign contributions; and reward investors and shareholders with generous returns on investment.

In 2022, Congress under the Biden administration, enacted the Inflation Reduction Act, which included provisions to reduce pharmaceutical costs for people with Medicare. The three significant features of the Act are: It lowers Medicare patients' maximum out-of-pockets costs from $3,000 per year to $2,000 per year. It caps the co-payment for insulin at $35 per month. And, for the very first time, the Act gave CMS permission to negotiate prices for ten drugs covered under Medicare. Although the Act benefits seniors, it did nothing to protect the rest of the public from high prescription drug costs and the Shkreli effect. Furthermore, drug manufactures and the U.S. Chamber of Commerce are taking the Biden administration to court, claiming Biden's actions to negotiate Medicare drug prices are unconstitutional.

## Private Equity

Private equity (PE) emerged with the 1980s wave of deregulation and preferential tax treatments, although it didn't find its way to healthcare until the early 2000s. Briefly, PE refers to limited private investment partnerships that buy and manage companies that are not publicly traded. Large pools of money, known as dry powder, which come from high net-worth individuals and institutional investors, are used to fund these deals. In two decades, "PE's investment in healthcare has increased twenty-fold from $5 billion in 2000 to $100 billion in 2018, with transactions growing from 78 to 855 within the same period."[13]

Although PE is an important source of capital for many parts of the healthcare system, it is an *investment.* It is loosely regulated, its transactions are hard to track, and its purpose is to maximize the investors' profits in a minimum amount of time, and then put the assets up for sale again. Unlike publicly traded companies, PE has very little oversight and is accountable primarily to its investors.[14] Since healthcare is a fragmented, $4.5 trillion dollars industry, rife with inefficiencies that is heavily supported by government subsidies, make it a very attractive investment, indeed.

Seeking quick returns on their investment and enabled by healthcare's significant fragmentation, PE's roll-up strategy—acquiring multiple small entities within the same sector and consolidating them into one entity—is a significant contributor to the market consolidation of nursing homes, hospices, air ambulances, physician practices, dialysis units, hospitals, and pain clinics, to name a few. PE is also a major investor in healthcare innovation including biopharmaceuticals, AI, and biotech.

While PE has penetrated all parts of the healthcare system, its investment in physician practices is a game changer. PE has surgically separated the clinical practice of medicine from the management of the practice, effectively putting a wall between the physicians' loyalty to patients and managements' loyalty to investors. Historically, state laws, to protect physician autonomy and safe-guard patient quality of care, have restricted the ownership of medical practices to physicians, only. However, with the promise of taking over the burdensome administrative responsibilities so physicians can focus on clinical care, PE legally separates the clinical practice of medicine from the management of a medical practice. The separation is clever, for it allows PE investors to work around the existing and long-standing state laws that prohibited corporate ownership of medical practices. Using this workaround, PE is investing heavily in medical practices that tend to be well reimbursed, such as dermatology and gastroenterology. PE is also investing heavily in hospice, and emergency departments and anesthesiology, specialties where surprise billing is common.

Claiming to reduce waste, PE's goal is to deliver a 20% to 30% return for their investors within five to seven years. Varying widely in how they pursue profits, typical methods include increasing prices, upcoding, doing procedures that aren't medically necessary, using protocols that increase patient visits, eliminating unprofitable services, reducing staff, and replacing highly trained staff with those with less training.[15]

Despite their claim that their for-profit investments make healthcare more affordable and accessible, evidence and precedent show a different bottom line. The result is not healthy for patients, physicians, nor the community. For patients, the typical painful effects are increased costs, more "surprise" bills, less quality, and poorer health outcomes. Physicians often find the management of their practice comes with the loss of clinical autonomy and extensive pressure to increase revenue and meet administrative targets, both of which cause moral distress and burnout.

However, the effect on the community is often the most severe. According to the Private Equity Stakeholder Project, "private equity owns about 486 U.S. hospitals, representing 8% of all private hospitals, 22% of all for-profit proprietary hospitals, and at least 26% of private equity owned hospitals serve rural communities."[16] Investing in hospitals is a good deal for investors but the consequences are born by staff and the community. Typically, the hospital is burdened by the purchase price, and often having to pay rent on the property it originally owned, the hospital is also loaded with excessive management fees, and the cost of management bonuses. Local control gives way to external control. In the name of efficiency, jobs are eliminated and the remaining staff is perpetually stressed by having to do more with less. Prices are raised, unprofitable services are discontinued—even services vital to the community, such as obstetrics and emergency care. Patients without insurance may be required to pay in advance for non-emergent tests and procedures, payments. In the worst case, some communities lose their hospitals, which means the community loses well-paying jobs and access to vital care, because closing the hospital is better for the investors' bottom line. The welfare of the community is simply an externalized cost.

PE is worrisome since it measures the value of a service in the size of the investors' profits, not in health outcomes. Although PE firms have been criticized for their luxurious profits at the expense of patients, physicians, and communities, like it or not, the U.S. healthcare system is a for-profit system. In 2019, national legislators proposed the "Stop Wall Street Looting Act," legislation to close regulatory, legal, and tax loopholes that make profits private and socializes costs.[17] Needless to say, the bill is still in committee, an action that implies the health of their constituents, which Congress is ethically bound to protect, isn't their first priority. Five years later, Massachusetts Senators Warren and Markley sponsored the Corporate Crimes Against Health Care Act of 2024. Aimed at preventing corporate and PE abuses in healthcare, the bill would hold PE firms and corporate executives accountable for actions that pushed healthcare entities into bankruptcy.[18]

In California, a group of emergency physicians and consumer advocate groups are suing to ban the split practice model, claiming the "investors pervasive direct and indirect control and/or influence over the medical practice, making decisions which bear directly and indirectly on the practice of medicine, rendering physicians as mere employees, and diminishing physician independence and freedom from commercial interests,"[19] violates anti-corporate medicine laws. The case goes to court in 2024.

Seeking quick returns on their investment, PE has penetrated all parts of the healthcare system. While it's most talked about effects—market consolidation, decreased competition, higher prices, and poorer quality—are important, equally important but less discussed is PE's disruption to the purpose of the healthcare system, a tacit shift from the production of health to the production of wealth.

## The Financialization of Healthcare

The financialization of healthcare refers to the pivot from making a profit from the production of health services to "the transformation of public, private, and corporate healthcare entities into salable and tradable assets from which the financial sector may accumulate capital."[20] Building on and going beyond the 1970s and 1980s privatization and corporatization of healthcare, financialization emerged in concert with the deregulation in the financial industry, the prioritization of shareholder value, the growth of private pools of unregulated capital, the relaxation of anti-trust legislation, and changes to Internal Revenue Service (IRS) rules that allowed non-profit hospitals to adopt for-profit strategies without tax liabilities. The growing entry of PE, investment banks, venture capital, and other types of investors into all aspects of healthcare has been a significant accelerant of financialization.

"Financialization captures the new forms of financial-sector ownership and control in the U.S. health care system, as well as the demands of financial markets for short-term profit growth and the distribution of this growth to financial actors that are *external* (italics added) to health care entities and U.S. households."[21] In short, any realized efficiencies benefit investors, only, whereas patients, healthcare employees, and communities bear the cost of these putative efficiencies.

In a working paper, Appelbaum, Blatt, and Cook describe the third stage of financialization as the dismantling of local healthcare systems. Rather than viewing local hospitals as a holistic system to provide patient care, financial investors view them as assets to buy and consolidate or buy and strip off the valuable services and then re-organize them into regional or national entities. These restructured holdings give investors more market power and economic leverage, as well as more local, state, and national legislative influence. Unfortunately, financially stressed hospitals have facilitated this process by selling to investors and by outsourcing ancillary units, like dietary and billing, as well as core services, like emergency, and anesthesiology. As a result, money is neither put back into hospital nor the community but flows out to the investors.[22]

The net result is greater systemic fragmentation and higher over-all costs, with less access and more health disparities for low-income patients and those living in already underserved geographic regions. This disruption further fragments the U.S. healthcare system along economic lines and portends that unprofitable population groups will receive fewer services unless further public subsidies can be found.

## Amazon

According to the American Hospital Association (AHA) report on disruption:

> Some of America's largest companies have made it their business to disrupt healthcare. And in 2019, six firms—Amazon, Apple, CVS Health/Aetna, Google/Alphabet, Walgreens, and Walmart—took significant steps to improve efficiency and make high-quality care more accessible. The moves they made are significant not because of their scale or size, but because they appear to be early indicators of the companies' longer-term ambitions in healthcare. The ramifications of these moves are likely to be felt in 2020 and beyond.[23]

Of the six firms, Amazon is one of the most ambitious. Until 2018, Amazon wasn't present in the healthcare market. Since then, it has introduced a handful of products. Some of them have failed. For instance, Haven, a not-for-profit joint venture created with Berkshire and JP Morgan Chase, was organized to provide high-quality low-cost healthcare for the three companies' employees and was disbanded in less than three years after its inception. Others, such as Pillpack, have already disrupted the pharmaceutical industry. Pillpack is a pharmacy fulfillment center. Working directly with the patients' doctors and insurers, Pillpack sends directly to the patient's door, a monthly "pack of pills" that are already pre-sorted by the day and time they are to be taken.

In 2022, Amazon made a bold move, launching Amazon Clinics in 32 states. Now in all 50 states, Amazon Clinics are a virtual healthcare service that offers treatment for about two dozen common, easy to treat health problems. The Clinic offers affordable, personalized care with no appointments by either video or live chat. After the message-based consultation, the patient received a personalized treatment plan that includes sending any prescriptions to the patient's preferred pharmacy. Upfront, patients are told the price of their care and pay in cash. The Clinic doesn't yet accept insurance, although insurance may cover pharmaceutical drug prescriptions.

The Clinic works directly with Amazon's digital and pharmacy assets. Designed to appeal to Generation Z and Millennials, half of whom don't have a primary care physician, the Clinic connects the patient to providers through the various telemedicine groups Amazon has partnered with. Although subject to intense regulatory scrutiny, Amazon is betting that primary care will become more digital. It is giving patients what they want: low-cost care that is convenient and accessible when and where they need it. With Amazon's 300 million customer base, strong supply chains, standardized, efficient processes, and cutting-edge technology, the Amazon Clinic has the potential to significantly disrupt and reshape the landscape of primary care.

**Retail Health**

Around 2000, retail health clinics began appearing in major pharmacy chains, like CVS and Walgreens, and in big box stores, like Walmart and Target. Although retail health is still in the experimental stage, the goal of retail clinics is to provide primary care at scale by making access to primary care as easy and convenient as grabbing a half gallon of milk. Usually open from 7 am to 7 pm seven days a week, retail clinics are generally staffed by NPs and physician assistants, who offer everything from treating minor health problems to preventive care to physicals. Accepting both cash and insurance, their prices are reliable, set, and posted on their websites. Retail care costs about 30% less than a doctor's office visit and about 80% less than an emergency department visit.

Research indicates that retail clinics make access to care easier and more affordable to patients. These clinics appeal to patients who don't have a primary care doctor, to uninsured patients, and to immigrants who don't speak English well. They are good choices for people who are young and relatively healthy. For other patients, retail clinics pose some challenges, including lack of care coordination, untimely referrals to specialists, over-utilization of laboratory and imaging services, and the risk that the problem was beyond the scope of the practitioner's training. Retail clinics with their convenience and affordability pose some challenges for the community.

By 2024, Walmart found disrupting primary care financially unsustainable. In 2019, Walmart deliberately entered the healthcare market with the "goal of becoming America's neighborhood health destination." Five years later, Walmart announced it would close its 51 Health Centers plus its virtual care services. Similarly, in 2024, Walgreens scaled back its primary care chain, closing its under-performing VillageMD clinics, or about half the clinics it opened between in the four-year period. Compared to Walmart, who closed all of its health centers, Walgreens kept its VillageMD clinics in regions with the greatest potential for profitability and growth.

For Walgreens, primary care clinics were only part of its business portfolio and closing under-performing clinics was part of a corporate cost-cutting move. Walmart, with its "goal of becoming America's neighborhood health destination," is a different story. On one hand, the story is about the challenges within the healthcare ecosystem that made it impossible for Walmart to succeed. First, as a cash business, there wasn't the volume at the right price to make it profitable. Second, for patients with insurance, Medicare and Medicaid don't cover the cost of care, and although commercial insurance pays more, its reimbursement for primary care is only slightly better than Medicare and Medicaid. Third, the revenue from referrals to specialty care and procedures went elsewhere, whereas, traditional providers use the more lucrative revenue from their specialty care to compensate for their low-paying primary care. Finally, labor shortages made recruiting difficult, and rising labor, drug, and supply costs out-paced the Health Centers' revenue.

The other part of the story is that retail health may not be a disruptor for affordable, easily accessible primary care. If Walmart with its significant resources, operational proficiencies, and its 4,630 stores—4,000 of which operate in the federal Health Services Research Administration's designated underserved areas—cannot operate primary care clinics profitably, the future of rural healthcare in America is ominous, indeed.[24,25]

## Vertical Integration

CVS Health is an example of retail health's potential for not just disrupting the delivery of healthcare but for also altering the historical configuration of the U.S. healthcare system. Billing itself as "America's leading health solutions company," CVS Health is more than an example of retail health disrupting the delivery of primary care by moving it out of the doctor's office and into the retail store, the patient's home, and the web. Following Mark Zuckerberg's maxim, "move fast and break things," CVS has vertically integrated physicians, national retail, or big-box stores, health insurance, pharmacy benefits management, and tech giants into a new and different healthcare ecosystem. By integrating provider and payer into one organization, CVS Health has disrupted the historical structure of the U.S. healthcare system. In short, CVS Health is poised to create a private version of "socialized medicine." Like the Veterans Administration healthcare where the government is both the payer and the provider, CVS Health is both the payer and the provider, albeit private.

CVS started in the 1960s as CVS, a pharmacy retail chain. It expanded to other sectors of the healthcare system in 2007, when it bought Caremark, which is one of the largest pharmacy benefit managers in the U.S. In 2018, CVS bought Aetna insurance, a merger that blurred the traditional lines between the insurer and the provider of prescription drugs. Then, in 2022, CVS Health bought the home health provider, Signify Health. It is now poised to purchase primary care physician practices to fulfill its primary care strategy.

These four purchases concentrate all aspects of a healthcare system into the hands of one, for-profit company. In contrast to the traditional, but fragmented,

U.S. healthcare system where its separate parts—physicians, prescription drugs, home health, and insurers—economically compete with each other, this vertical integration gives CVS Health the capacity to coordinate and standardize the interaction among the four groups. The ability to nationally standardize medical treatment protocols; control access to prescription drugs, tests, specialists, and surgery; and direct the location of care to the home, the hospital, or a virtual location signify that healthcare is no longer a cottage industry where physicians practice according to local standards and where they were trained. This kind of control, coordination, and national presence, which gives CVS Health tremendous financial and market share advantage, has the potential to move care out of the hospital and into the home. This will further lessen physicians' influence in the delivery of care and increase the economic fragility of many local, independent hospitals.

CVS Health is one of many national healthcare giants that are building vertically integrated systems. Because of their national scope and financial strength, most other healthcare organizations—especially smaller ones—will be unable to compete. Although poised to significantly revolutionize the U.S. healthcare system, it is too early to tell whether these vertically integrated corporations will make healthcare more accessible and affordable for many or more profitable for a few. It's unknown whether these new corporations will pass their cost savings on to patients or reward stockholders with higher dividends.

Precedent, however, shows that the patient has consistently suffered to the benefit of the share-holder. Moreover, there's clear agreement that the current trends in consolidation and vertical integration drive up hospital prices by as much as 30%.[26] It's too early to know what will happen to small rural hospitals. Will they pass away like small town retail stores did when the big box stores came to town? It's too early to know the effect of redirecting care into the home. On one hand, with the current staffing shortages, some hospitals may welcome the redirection of care away from the hospital; others may rue the loss of profitable care. On the other hand, redirection of care into the home puts the cost of care on to families—someone has to stay home from work to do what hospital nurses and others used to do. Based on previous experience, it can be safely assumed that this new, vertically integrated ecosystem will simply increase profits for a few stakeholders and probably worsen health outcomes. What is known is that other big businesses are busy creating their version of the CVS Health model.

## Double-Edged Swords

Disruptors, like telemedicine and retail health, are double-edged sword. On one hand, these disruptors have the capacity to make healthcare more accessible, convenient, and more affordable. On the other hand, the current trend for telehealth and retail health is the prioritization of economic growth over quality. Both disruptors raise concerns about data privacy, continuity of care, and care coordination.

With an increasing number of Americans having multiple chronic diseases, care coordination is a particular concern. About 42% of the population must coordinate care between two specialists and 12% have five or more chronic diseases, which means at least five specialists are involved in their care. If telehealth and retail health are part of a large system with an integrated electronic health record, a patient who needs follow-up care can see their personal physician, who immediately has access to the relevant details of the visit. However, when the visit is with a stand-alone company, records don't easily transfer and the patient is responsible for coordinating his own care. The risk for telehealth and retail patients who don't have a relationship with a primary care physician is healthcare becomes a DIY enterprise with the patient responsible for coordinating his own care.

### Horizontal Consolidation

Horizontal consolidation refers to mergers of hospitals with other hospitals, physician practices with similar practices, and insurers with insurers. Hospitals began consolidating in the 1990s to gain economies of scale and to increase revenue through greater market power to leverage greater reimbursement from commercial insurers. The effect on what was once a cottage industry has been noticeable. According to the AHA, there were 6,120 hospitals in the U.S. in 2024, of which 5,129 were community hospitals.[27] Of these community hospitals, 68% are part of a hospital system.[28]

Horizontal consolidation of hospitals is expected to continue. Consolidation provides access to intellectual and financial capital, as well as access to new markets, technology, and innovation. Due to Medicare's poor reimbursement, becoming part of a large hospital system, which gives them access to financial capital, larger markets, and better negotiating leverage with private insurers, is especially important to hospitals with larger Medicare populations. Seemingly, this is a win-win. The smaller hospitals gain financial stability and the larger hospitals gain more patients. The sicker patients are steered to the larger hospitals within the system, since care is coordinated within the hospital system.

Horizontal consolidation does not change the structure of the healthcare. The downside of horizontal consolidation is it is a perturbation, further distressing an unhealthy system for it's put smaller hospitals at a competitive disadvantage. Hospital consolidation has also shifted strategic and financial decisions from local to corporate control. Thus, decisions, such as layoffs and reductions to service lines, once the purview of a local hospital board, are now made in corporate offices where the impact on the local economy and on people's health is neither seen nor felt.

As a result, the Federal Trade Commission (FTC) has increased its scrutiny over mergers and acquisitions on the grounds of public interest. Certainly, protecting the public's healthcare needs is important; however, antitrust scrutiny ignores the root causes of consolidation. Antitrust scrutiny will not solve the public's concerns about equity, rising costs, and access to care, which are generated by structure. In fact, as Ken Kaufman points out, more scrutiny squeezes hospitals between "two hard and conflicting realities:"

> The first reality is that partnerships will continue to be a necessary and critical part of healthcare strategy, particularly as financial performance and

patient access continue to be pervasive and ongoing problems for hospitals. The second reality is that antitrust enforcement will continue to create strong barriers to these same partnerships that are necessary for both provider stability and overall community well-being.[29]

## Vertical Integration Changes the Structure of Healthcare

Horizontal consolidation does not change the structure of the healthcare system, whereas, vertical integration does. Vertical integration refers to uniting the financing and the delivery of care into a cooperative whole within one organization. Not all integrated companies are the same and there's a mix of old and new players. Founded in 1945, Kaiser Permanente is the oldest and is known for its low-cost, high-quality care. Billing itself a managed care consortium, Kaiser owns and operates hospitals, employs its physicians, and offers prepaid health plans and insurance. Kaiser Permanente, essentially, functions as a universal healthcare system. In contrast, CVS and UnitedHealthcare Group are new players that have integrated different parts of the fragmented U.S. healthcare system to fit their unique business goals. CVS offers health insurance, employs physicians, has its own pharmacy, and delivers primary care through its walk-in clinics. UnitedHealthcare Group offers health insurance, employs physicians, has its own pharmacy benefits management, provides data analytics, and over 8,000 hospitals are in its network.

With vertical integration, healthcare is no longer a cottage industry and physicians are no longer entrepreneurs but employees. In the U.S., vertical integration, because it is a piecemeal phenomenon, further accentuates the problems of an already fragmented system. First, vertical integration tacitly gives the insurer more control over the utilization of care, or in other words, the practice of medicine, which is instrumental in controlling costs. Second, vertical integration has not made healthcare more affordable or accessible. Patients still need insurance to access care. However, vertical integration restricts patients' choices, directing patients to the hospitals, physicians, and pharmacies the insurance covers. While good for business, perhaps, not so good for patients. Costs for patients haven't decreased, but their quality of care is often worse.

Ironically, peer countries' universal healthcare system also integrates the financing and delivery of care into one system. The differences are significant, however. In the U.S. access to and type of care are determined by the type of insurance one has; in peer countries, everyone has access and to the same kinds of care. Peer countries have tightly regulated, non-profit insurance; whereas, we have for-profit insurance based on market dynamics.

Finally, as a scattershot endeavor, vertical integration adds to the fragmentation of the U.S. healthcare system. According to Paul Keckley:

> The fragmentation in U.S. healthcare is recognized inside the industry's board rooms and C suites, but short-term strategies to avoid risk supersede long-term actions toward systemness. Scenario plans by healthcare's insiders reflect incremental changes in the industry while outsiders like Big Tech

see transformational changes. They develop system platform solutions applicable to many industries while healthcare develops solutions specific to sectors wanting protection from outsiders and infidels who dare challenge their status quo.[30]

## Disruption and Decision Points

Healthcare has been disrupted by market consolidation and new players entering the market, such as retail health, NPs, and digital technology (Figure 4.1). Despite the consolidation, the disruptors have not altered the structure of the healthcare system.

According to systems thinking, a decision point refers to a point in time where a decision about which action to take needs to be made. Decision points are identified by a diverging pathway or the emergence of alternative options. Finances and technology have long been the twin drivers of healthcare consolidation and innovation; however, COVID-19 also played a role. Hospitals that were vertically integrated—had their own insurance products, employed their own physicians, and had their own pharmacy benefits management—did better financially than other hospitals.

Generally speaking, hospital systems, insurers, and physician practices have gained economic and competitive advantages with vertical and horizontal consolidation. However, new markets and consolidation are self-protective. Not surprisingly, different stakeholders have different perspectives. For instance, a 2023, special report from the AHA regarding seven large companies disrupting healthcare stated: "[t]hey all share some common goals: to improve access, care coordination and make care more affordable as consumers *take greater responsibility for their own health*" (italics added).[31] On the other hand, a February, 2024 KFF poll showed that about 75% of surveyed adults worried about affording unexpected medical bills and the cost of healthcare, in general.[32]

The question is the best way to go forward. How do we, as Americans, construct a healthy healthcare system: one that's efficient, effective, and equitable?

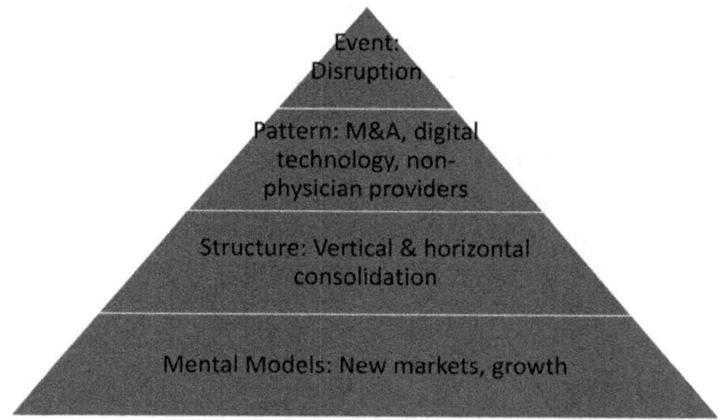


*Figure 4.1* Iceberg Model: Disruptors

One that includes all Americans? Although it has been piecemeal and involves organizations that have market power and cash reserves, vertical integration has shown that costs can be controlled by integrating insurers, hospitals, doctors, and pharmaceutical benefits. While vertical integration is quietly restructuring the U.S. healthcare system, it further fragments an already fragmented system. Vertical integration excludes the patients who don't live in higher income regions as well as the organizations that don't have the resources to compete in a market designed to benefit the strongest stakeholders.

Because the mental models of healthcare as a cottage industry no longer apply, and because the contemporary structural changes—financialization, horizontal consolidation, and vertical integration—indicate that the U.S. healthcare system is morphing, this is a good time for Americans to examine their values and priorities around the purpose of the U.S. healthcare system. As Americans, we have a choice. The public can be passive and remain silent, allowing the powerful stakeholders to continue the restructuring of healthcare to meet their needs. We can react out of habit and fear, causing our brains to block novel information, prevent new connections with others, and be blind to alternate possibilities, all in support of the status quo. Or, we can advocate for a new and more holistic structure that is more effective, efficient, and fair, and includes everyone.

## Questions for the Reader

The questions provide an opportunity to examine your own mental models and values and to imagine other stakeholders' beliefs, fears, and values.

1 Do health insurance and pharmaceutical drugs cost too much? If so, who should control their costs—the government, the market? What are the upsides and downsides of your choice? What might others think?
2 Knowing that insurers negotiate drug prices through pharmacy benefit managers and the federal government negotiates drug prices for the VA, do you think the federal government should negotiate Medicare drug prices? Why do you believe this; what might others think?
3 If your insurance insisted that a family member be cared for at home, in what ways might home care burden or benefit your family?
4 Do you and your family have a primary care physician? If not, why not?
5 Have you, or someone you know, used telehealth, a health app, or a retail clinic? If yes, what did you like and didn't like about the experience? Did you get the expected results? Was it worth the cost? Should your physician be paid the same for a telehealth visit as for an in-office visit?
6 If available, would you, or someone you know, seek healthcare at a retail location? Would price make a difference? What are the pluses and minuses of retail health and for whom?
7 Did your hospital have a negative profit margin in 2022? Is your hospital currently financially stable? What would happen to you and your family if your hospital were to eliminate some services or close its doors?

8 If you needed a non-emergent service from your hospital, could you pay for it ahead of time? If you couldn't, how might this affect your health? While pre-payment is a good business decision for hospitals, is this ethical? Why; what might others think?
9 Should the purpose of U.S. healthcare system be a saleable and tradeable asset from which the financial sector makes short-term profits, or should the purpose of U.S. healthcare system be to produce health for all Americans? Who are the winners and losers with the financialization of healthcare? What might others think?
10 Whom do you trust to make healthcare more affordable for everyone: Big Tech, private corporations, the federal government, market forces, no one? Why; what might others think?
11 Whom do you trust to determine what tests, procedures, drugs you need, and what specialists you should see? Your doctor, your insurance company, the government? Why; what might others think?
12 What is your solution for making the U.S. healthcare system more affordable? Making it more convenient? What might others think?

## Notes

1 Over 77% of physicians are employed. (2024, April 16). *Advisory Board.* https://www.advisory.com/daily-briefings/2024/04/16.
2 Savard, I., Al Hakim, G., & Kilpatrick, K. (2022, December 17). The added value of the nurse practitioner: An evolutionary concept analysis. *National Center for Biotechnology Information.* https://www.ncbi.nlm.nih.gov/pmc/articles/PMC10006655.
3 Morgan, P.A., Smith, V.A., Berkowitz, T.S.C., Edelman, D., Van Houtven, C.H., Woolson, S.L., et al. (2019, June). Impact of physicians, nurse practitioners, and physician assistants on utilization and costs for complex patients. *Health Affairs.* https://www/healthaffairs.org/doi/10.1377/hlthaff.2019.0014.
4 Robeznieks, A. (2022, March 17). Amid doctor shortage NPs and PAs seem like a fix. Data's in: Nope. *AMA.* https//:www.ama-assn.org/practice-management/scope.
5 Robeznieks, A. (2022, March 17). Amid doctor shortage NPs and PAs seem like a fix. Data's in: Nope. AMA. https//:www.ama-assn.org/practice-management/scope.
6 Greenwood, H., Krzyzaniak, N., Peiris, R., Clark, J., Scott, A.M., Cardona, M., Griffith, R., & Glasziou, P. (2022, March 11). Telehealth Versus Face-to-face Psychotherapy for Less Common Mental Health Conditions: Systematic Review and Meta-analysis of Randomized Controlled Trials. *PubMed.* https://pubmed.ncbi.nlm.nih/gov/35475081.
7 Digital Health – United States. *Statista Market Forecast.* https://www.statistica.com/outlook/hmo/digital-health/united-states.
8 *Statista.* (2023, September 12). Prescription drug expenditure U.S. 1960–2021. https://statista.com/statistics/184914/.
9 Kurani, N., Cotliar, D., & Fox, C. (2022, February 8). How Do Prescription Drug Costs in the United States Compare with Other Countries. *Peterson-KFF Health System Tracker.* https://www.healthsystemtracker.org/chart.
10 Hamel, L., Lopez, L., Kerzinger, A. et al. (2022, October 20). Public Opinion on Prescription Drugs and Their Prices. *KFF.* https://www.kff.org/health-costs/poll-finding.
11 Schlanger, Z. (2015, September 21). Martin Shkreli on Raising Price of AIDS Drug, 5,000 percent: "I Think Profits Are a Great Thing." *Newsweek.* https:// www.newsweek.com/martin-shkreli-d.
12 News: Chairman Sanders Releases Report Exposing How Weight Loss Drugs Could Bankrupt American Healthcare. (2024, May 15). www.Sanders.gov/press-releases/news/chairman-sanders-releases.

13 Mathews, W., & Roxas, R. (2022, May 13). Private equity and its effect on patients: a window into the future. *International Journal of Health Economics and Management.* www.ncbi.nlm.nih.gov/pmc/articles/PMC9125965/.
14 Olson, Laura Katz. (2022). *Ethically Challenged: Private Equity Storms US Health Care*. Baltimore: Johns Hopkins University Press.
15 Scheffler, R.M., Alexander, L., Fulton, B.D., Arnold, D.R., & Abdelhadi, O.A. (2023, July 10). Monetizing Medicine: Private Equity and Competition in Physician Practice Markets. *Berkley Public Health.* https://publichealth.berkley.edu/news/media
16 PESP Hospital Tracker. Private Equity Stakeholder Project. https://pestakeholder.org/private-equity-hospital-tracker.
17 Warren, Baldwin, Brown, Pocan, Jayapal, Colleagues. https://www.waren.senate.gov/newsroom/press.
18 Warren, E. (2024, June 11). Senators Warren and Markley introduce the corporate crimes against health care act of 2024. *News Release*. https://www.warren.senate.gov/press.
19 Wolfson, B.J. (2022, December 22). ER doctors call private equity practices illegal and seek to ban them. *Kaiser Health News*. https://kffhealthnews.org/article/er-doctors
20 Bruch, J.D., Roy, V., & Grogan, C.M. (2024, January 11). The financialization of Health in the United States. *New England Journal of Medicine.* 390 (2) 178–182.
21 Bruch, J.D., Roy, V., & Grogan, C.M. (2024, January 11). The financialization of Health in the United States. *New England Journal of Medicine.* 390 (2) 178–182.
22 Applebaum, E., Batt, R., & Cook, A. (2021, September 9). Working Paper: Financialization in health care: The transformation of U.S. hospital systems. *Center for Economic and Policy Research.* https://cepr.net/report/working-paper.
23 American Hospital Association. (2023, February 14). Special Report: How 7 Disruptors Will Transform Hospitals in 2023. https://www.aha.org/aha-center-health-innovation
24 Landi, H. (2024, April 30). Walmart's Health shutdown underscores under-scores major challenges for health 'disruptors.' Retail health disruptors. *Fierce Healthcare*. https://www.fiercehealthcare.com/providers/walmart.
25 Kaufman, Ken. (2024, May 22). Walmart's primary care failure is important and a problem. *Thoughts from Ken Kauffman.* https://www.kauffmanhall.com/insights/thoughts-ken.
26 Beaulieu, N.D., Chernew, M.E., McWilliams, J., et al. (2023, January 24/31). Organization and Performance of US Health Systems. *JAMA*. 329 (4) 325–335. https://jamanetwork.com/journals/jama/fullar.
27 Fast Facts on US Hospitals, 2024. (2024, January 12). *AHA.* https://www.aha.org/statistics/fast-facts-us-hospitals.
28 Fast Facts on US Hospitals, 2024. (2024, January 12). *AHA.* https://www.aha.org/system/files/media/file/2024/.
29 Kaufman, K. (2024, June 20). The state of play in health care antitrust reinforcement. *Kaufman Hall*. https://kaufmanhall.com/insights/thoughts-ken.
30 The Keckley Report-Paul Keckley. (2023, January 30). Big Tech Advantage in Healthcare... https://paulkeckley.com/the-keckley-report.
31 Special Report: How 7 Disruptors Will Transform Health Care in 2023. (2023, February 14). *The American Hospital Association*. https://www.aha.org/aha-center-health-innovation.
32 KFF Health Tracking Poll February 2024: Votes on Two Key Health Care Issues: Affordability and ACA. (2024, February 21). https://www.kff.org//affordable-care-act/poll.

# 5 Effectiveness

## The Value of Systemic Effectiveness

Healthy people are the backbone of a healthy country. Healthy people are economically productive and important to national security. Healthy people feel better, live longer, have more energy, are more productive, and are active participants in the lives of their families and communities. Overall, healthy people have a better quality of life. Access to an effective healthcare system is important to being healthy.

The purpose of a healthcare system is to produce health. The effectiveness of any system is measured by the degree it successfully produces its product. In this case, the effectiveness of a nation's healthcare system is determined by its ability to produce healthy citizens. But, what is health? There isn't a universally accepted definition of health. The word doesn't evoke a consistent image in the minds of stakeholders. It's often assumed that health means the same to you as it does to me, the same to the insurer as it does to the patient, the same to the young as the old, and the same to those with life-threatening diseases as it does to those with chronic diseases.

There are many definitions of health; however, three have had long-term sticking power. One common definition is health is the absence of disease. This is a derivative of the 19th-century definition of biomedicine: "the science of diagnosing, treating, curing, and preventing disease." Most medical schools still use this definition. Another is "health is the capacity to work." This early 20th- century definition is attributed to Frederick T. Gates, the chief lieutenant for John D. Rockefeller Sr.'s financial empires and philanthropies.[1] The third definition is the 1948 definition promulgated by the World Health Organization (WHO): "Health is a state of complete physical, mental, and social well-being, not just the absence of disease."

Without a standardized definition of health, a plethora of surrogate measures are used to evaluate the performance of a healthcare system. These measures fall into two large categories: quality and safety. The most basic measure of quality is health outcomes and the most basic measure for safety is preventable harm from medical errors.

The effectiveness of the U.S. healthcare system is evaluated against national standards and against international standards and data. National measures and national comparisons allow physicians, hospitals, large hospital systems, and policymakers to evaluate and compare the quality and safety of medical care against

DOI: 10.4324/9781003538226-6

a variety of private and public U.S. benchmarks. International standards and data compare health outcomes of the U.S. healthcare system to that of other countries, usually similar wealthy countries.

## The Quality Chasm: National Quality and Safety Comparison Data

Ask any American and most will tell you that America has the best healthcare system in the world. Despite grumbling about healthcare costs, most claim that the quality of care is better in the U.S. than in any other country. Unfortunately, by almost every measure the U.S. healthcare system is not nearly as effective as other countries' healthcare systems. About twenty-five years ago, the Institute of Medicine (IOM) released a landmark report, "To Error is Human: Building a Safer Healthcare System."[2] Stating that as many as 98,000 people die annually in American hospitals from errors that could have been prevented, the report shocked the nation with its finding. To put the 98,000 deaths in perspective, medical errors then caused more deaths annually than did motor vehicle accidents or breast cancer. Yet, the Hippocratic oath states, "first do no harm."

In the following twenty-five years, those statistics haven't improved. Today, medical errors are considered the third leading cause of death.[3] Asserting that healthcare was at least a decade behind other industries, such as the airline industry, in assuring basic safety, the IOM report called for systemic change. The report asserted that medical errors and poor health outcomes were not caused by "bad" people but by "bad" systems. The IOM report specifically cited fragmentation, faulty, and overly complex processes baked into the delivery of care.

A few years later, the IOM released another report, "Crossing the Quality Chasm,"[4] which called for a fundamental redesign of the American healthcare system. Stating that the American healthcare system "harms too frequently and routinely fails to deliver its potential benefits,"[5] the report recommended sweeping systemic changes to improve the safety and quality of care delivered by the U.S. healthcare system.

Both IOM reports caught the attention of policymakers, healthcare leaders, insurers, regulators, and some of the public. Since the early 2000s, numerous national private and public organizations are involved in evaluating and improving the quality and safety of care in the U.S. Two national organizations deserve special mention. One is The Joint Commission (TJC), a private, non-profit organization. Founded in 1951, the TJC is the nation's oldest accrediting body, certifying that hospitals meet quality and safety requirements for receiving Medicare and Medicaid reimbursement. The other is the Centers for Medicare and Medicaid Services (CMS). It is the largest insurer in the U.S., providing Medicare for seniors, Medicaid for the qualified poor, Children's Health Insurance Program (CHIPS) for children of qualified low-income families.

Since it provides insurance coverage for about 40% of the U.S. population, CMS is, understandably, interested in assuring it is paying for high-quality care. Quality is defined as care that is safe, timely, effective, efficient, equitable, and patient-centered, often referred to as STEEEP. CMS collects a large variety of data from a wide variety of healthcare delivery settings and uses the data in its quality improvement, payment incentive, and Star Rating programs. The Star Rating program helps patients choose and compare hospitals based on their quality of care—mortality, safety, readmission, timeliness, effectiveness, and patient experience. Ratings range from one to five stars, with five being the best. Patients can access any hospital's rating on the website https://hospitalcompare.io.

## Twenty Years of Improvement Efforts Yield Mixed Results

Twenty plus years of widespread and continuous efforts to improve the quality and safety of the U.S. healthcare system have yielded mixed results. While some significant and positive results have narrowed the quality chasm, progress has been mixed and too many people still suffer from harmful events. Wrong leg amputated, wrong medicine given, wrong patient disconnected from the ventilator, lethal falls, infected surgical sites, poorly coordinated care, and inaccurate diagnosis are still too common.

Reporting on quality and safety data from 2000 to 2022, the Agency for Healthcare Research and Quality (AHREQ) found that of the 176 measures used to evaluate hospital quality and safety 43.8% improved, 48.8% stayed the same, and 7.4% worsened.[6] The data also showed significant health disparities. Health disparities are the differences in health outcomes that are linked to racial, ethnic, and economic disadvantages. These disparities tend to significantly vary by region of the U.S. Generally speaking, quality is worse in the southeastern U.S. compared to other regions.

Reflecting on 20 years of work to improve the quality and safety of the U.S. healthcare system, Mark Chassin, MD, one of the authors of the original report noted three broad areas for monitoring and improvement: (1) medical errors, (2) overuse of unnecessary and/or low value tests and treatments, and (3) missed opportunities to give effective care.[7]

## International Quality Comparison Data

Every country's healthcare system is unique and no one system is perfect. Healthcare systems vary in their strengths and weaknesses and, as to be expected, they vary in their effectiveness. It's well known that the U.S. has the most expensive healthcare system in the world. It's not so well known, however, that compared with systems of similar wealthy nations, the effectiveness of the U.S. healthcare system falls painfully short, with its lower life expectancy and highest death rates for treatable conditions.

Generally speaking, the rule of thumb to measure the effectiveness of a country's healthcare system is whether the average citizen is able to lead a long, healthy, and productive life. By these metrics, the U.S. healthcare system falls short. Falling short has significantly worsened since the 1980s, according to reports from the Organization for Economic and Cooperative Development (OECD), the Kaiser Family Foundation (KFF), and the Commonwealth Fund (CF).

The KFF and the CF are well respected for their international healthcare comparison work. Both use international data supplied by the OECD and the WHO.

In 2021 and 2023, the CF and the KFF, respectively, released international comparison reports. The CF report was titled "Mirror, Mirror 2021—Reflecting Poorly: Health Care in the U.S. Compared to other High-Income Countries,"[8] and the KFF was titled, "How Does the Quality of the U.S. Health Care System Compare to Other Countries"?[9] Both reports compared the U.S. healthcare system with similar, wealthy countries, although the CF report restricted its comparison to ten other countries: Australia, Canada, France, Germany, Netherland, New Zealand, Norway, Sweden, Switzerland, and the United Kingdom. Using the same ten countries, the KFF report also included Japan and a few other western European countries. Significantly, both reports showed that the U.S. lags behind peer countries in health outcomes.

### The U.S. Has the Lowest Average Life Expectancy

Life expectancy is a projection, estimating the average number of years that a person can expect to live. The most common measure is life expectancy at birth. The measure is affected by gender, age, race, and geographic location. Life expectancy is an important and basic measure of the effectiveness of a healthcare system and commonly used for national and international comparisons.

Compared to similar wealthy countries, the U.S. has the lowest average life expectancy, 76 years, compared to peer countries' 80 years, a number that has been gradually dropping in the U.S. since 2014. Average doesn't tell the full story; however, because life expectancy varies by current age, race, ethnicity, gender, income, and geography. According to 2021, Centers for Disease Control and Prevention (CDC) data, average life expectancy in the U.S. is 76 years; but it is 70.8 years for African Americans and 65.2 years for Native Americans, and it's 78.6 years for Hispanics.[10] Average life span for Hawaiians is 80.7 years, but it's only 71.9 years for Mississippians.[11]

The years between 2020 and 2022 registered the largest, two-year drop in life expectancy in a very long time. The drop was attributed to opioid abuse, economic disparity, suicide, and obesity, as well as the U.S. having more COVID-19 deaths than peer countries. Compared to its peers, the U.S. has the highest suicide rate; its death rate from physical assault it seven times greater than its peers; and the U.S. obesity rate is almost twice that of its peers.

### The U.S. Ranks High in the Number of Avoidable Deaths

Avoidable deaths are another contributor to the U.S. having the lowest life expectancy. Avoidable deaths are a tacit measure of the healthiness of the average citizen. These are deaths that occur at a younger age and from causes that are preventable and treatable. Basically, avoidable deaths are deaths that might have been avoided with timely access to effective healthcare. Avoidable deaths include unmanaged hypertension, heart disease, unmanaged diabetes, and some cancers. Since 2015, avoidable deaths have been rising in the U.S., with the U.S. having a higher rate than many of its peers. According to 2021, OECD data, the U.S. preventable deaths at 265 per 100,000 population are higher than the OECD average of 199 per 100,000 population and much higher than the OECD best performer average of 97 avoidable deaths per 100,000 population.[12]

U.S. adults are much more likely to have multiple chronic diseases than adults living in other wealthy countries. According to CDC data, about 60% of American adults have one chronic disease, about 40% have two or more, and about 11% have three or more chronic health conditions. According to CDC data, adults with multiple chronic diseases have a poorer quality of life and an increased risk of early death compared with healthy adults. In the U.S., the prevalence of chronic disease varies widely by geography region, with a higher concentration in the southeast. People of Color and low economic status are also associated with a greater prevalence of chronic diseases.

Although chronic diseases are a leading cause of avoidable deaths, research shows that a substantial portion of these deaths are attributed to a handful of modifiable risk factors. These factors are typically grouped into three categories: (1) lifestyle factors, such as weight control, exercise, smoking cessation, social connections, and alcohol in moderation; (2) disease management such as blood pressure, cholesterol, and blood sugar control; and (3) preventive screenings, such as colonoscopies and mammograms.

While many people with chronic diseases can lead full and healthy lives, to do so requires support and ongoing medical attention. Diabetes is a case in point. Amputation of toes, feet, and lower legs is a risk factor for diabetics, and lower-extremity amputation is a risk factor for premature death. The risks of lower extremity amputation vary by race, geography, and socioeconomic status; however, the risk is higher for African and Native Americans and those living in rural areas where access to healthcare is limited.

The irony is painful. Despite the well-known fact that avoidable deaths are, well, avoidable, the U.S. healthcare system continues to be designed to emphasize acute, episodic treatment instead of prevention and coordinated management of chronic diseases. Furthermore, many patients don't know that preventive services—such as mammograms and colonoscopies—are ACA-required covered benefits without co-pays. However, due to the *Braidwood vs Becerra* some preventive services now require co-pays. Because of this lawsuit, a judge in the North District Court of Texas ruled that some of the ACA's requirements regarding payment of preventive services without co-pays were unconstitutional and violated religious rights, and the court also imposed limits on the government's ability to enforce these requirements. While some states have enacted legislation to protect payment of preventive care without co-pays, others have not.

Whether it's a design flaw in the U.S. healthcare system or something else, evidence shows that the "U.S. health disadvantage persists even when the comparison was limited to the most advantaged groups: people in the highest socioeconomic bracket, white, insured, and without a history of tobacco use, drinking, or obesity."[13] In other words, the health status of wealthy White Americans is better than that of the average American but not as good as the health status of the average citizen in other wealthy countries.[14]

### The U.S. Has the Highest Infant and Maternal Mortality Rates

The U.S. infant and maternal deaths are more than triple the rate of most of its peers. For a long time, U.S. women have had the highest rate of maternal mortality due to complications of pregnancy and childbirth. A third of these deaths occur at the time of birth; however, a full half of them occur within one year of giving birth. Racial disparities play a role, with the maternal death rate for Black women 2.5 times greater than for White women and 3 times greater than Hispanic women. Other factors include the U.S.'s high rate of Cesarean deliveries, birth-related infections, inadequate postpartum care, and socioeconomic inequalities that contribute to chronic diseases like heart disease, obesity, and diabetes. Significantly, across the U.S. there's an alarming lack of maternity care—36% of U.S. counties don't have obstetric services and 55% of rural hospitals do not provide obstetric care.

Infant mortality is the death of an infant within the first year of life. Infant mortality is an important measure of the effectiveness of a country's healthcare system, reflecting unhealthy *in utero* and postnatal conditions. Although infant mortality rates have declined slightly in all wealthy countries for the past 15 years or so, the decline has been greater in peer countries. In 2022, the U.S. rate was 5.5 deaths per 1,000 live births, compared to the German rate of 2.1 deaths per 1,000 live births.[15] In the U.S., the infant mortality rate varies widely by race—the death rate of White babies is 4.49 compared to the death rate of Black babies at 10.6 deaths per 1,000 live births.[16] Infant mortality rate also varies by geography with a death rate of 8.6 in Mississippi compared to roughly 3 per 1,000 live births in New Hampshire.[17]

Also, compared to its peers the U.S. has the second worst rates of low-birth weight infants and premature births. Both are indicators of unhealthy *in utero* and prenatal conditions. Precedent and evidence indicate that the high mortality rates and low birth weight babies reflects lifestyle and social factors, as well as the effectiveness of the healthcare system.

### The U.S. Has a High Burden of Disease

Burden of disease is a more sophisticated measure of health outcomes than morbidity alone. Burden of disease takes into account the years of life lost to early death and the years of poor health due to disease, injury, and disability. Measured in terms of disability adjusted life years (DALY), it is a standardized measure that calculates the effects of mortality and morbidity in a population. Mortality refers to death. Morbidity refers to the state of not being healthy because of the presence of a disease, injury, or disability. One DALY represents the loss of one year of good health. The higher the score, the greater the burden of disease. In short, burden of disease is a measure of years of life lost due to premature deaths and poor health in populations that allows for comparisons of morbidities across countries, between different populations, and over time.

Chronic diseases are a primary cause of poor health. Since the 1990s, the prevalence of chronic diseases in American children and young adults has grown. The good news is that since the 2000s, the burden of disease has declined in both the U.S. and peer countries. However, the U.S. has a higher age-adjusted DALY rate than its peers. According to 2019 data, the U.S. had the highest DALY rate of 26,061 per 100,000 population, compared with the average rate of 18,987 per 100,000 population. Japan had the lowest, at a DALY rate of 15,866 per 100,000 population.[18]

The measure is well named: *burden* of disease. Burden refers to the economic and psycho-social costs of premature death and poor health. These costs are born by patients, their families, and by society at large. From the patients' perspective, *burden* is associated with direct and indirect economic costs, such as lost wages, expensive medical bills, risk of losing a job and health insurance, economic hardships, and increased risk of medical bankruptcy. The economic costs to society are also great, including the direct costs of medical care and indirect costs of lost productivity, lost talent and creativity, lost tax revenue, as well as the costs of increased social services and benefits for families of the ill and deceased.

Although more difficult to measure, the psychosocial burden of premature death and poor health on families is also enormous. Ineluctably, premature death and poor health cause every family member to suffer, each in his own way. Patients lose valued familiar roles, self-image, and a familiar lifestyle. Family members are also burdened by the loss of familiar roles and lifestyle, as well as the burden of extra work for the healthy spouse or care giver, more social isolation, and the greater risk among family members of depression, anxiety, and guilt, and other symptoms of emotional stress.

Because burden of disease allows for comparisons of morbidities across countries, between different populations within a country, and over time, the burden of disease data helps policymakers evaluate the effectiveness of the healthcare system from multiple perspectives. Knowing which diseases are prevalent in which populations and whether some populations carry a greater burden than others are two perspectives that are indicators are of the system's global effectiveness. For instance, diabetes disproportionately affects Native Americans, racial and ethnic minorities, and low-income adults. And, it's about twice as prevalent in the "diabetes belt," which reaches across the southeastern states and up into Appalachia, and elsewhere. Researchers attribute the prevalence to a variety of factors, including socioeconomic status, lifestyle factors, environmental conditions, availability of healthy foods and physical activity, and access to healthcare.

A second perspective regarding burden of disease is whether the right resources, in the right amounts are at the right location. For instance, the high prevalence of maternal deaths in the U.S. is associated with the lack of access to maternity care and that women of color are under treated compared with White women are two examples of resource problems. That there's higher incidence of lower limb amputations with diabetics living in southeastern states than diabetics living elsewhere is a negative example of the right resources at right location.

Cost-benefit analysis, which is another perspective of effectiveness, measures whether the outcome is worth the cost. For example, data show that the cost of screening many people for colon cancer is more beneficial, or less expensive, than treating colon cancer in a few. Finally, burden of disease data shows "which burdens and whose burdens matter." This perspective illuminates the influence of social values and prior policy decisions on health outcomes. The HIV epidemic exemplifies "which burdens and whose burdens mattered." It took about five years before significant resources were spent on understanding the virus and treating those infected by the HIV virus, because the epidemic started in and was, seemingly, confined to gay males. On the flip side, in the summer of 2014, 17 million people uploaded videos of themselves taking the "Ice Bucket Challenge" a fund-raiser that dramatically increased awareness about amyloid lateral sclerosis, an uncommon disease that affects the nervous system. In less than six weeks an unprecedented $115 million was raised, accelerating the research against the disease.

These four perspectives regarding burden of disease data provide reliable information for evaluating the effectiveness of the U.S. healthcare system. Used together they provide a comprehensive picture of the distribution of diseases, the distribution of healthcare's resources for treatment, and the effectiveness of healthcare policy regarding the distribution of resources. These four perspectives also provide valuable information for prescribing future, systemic health policies and interventions.

## The U.S. Ranks Last in the Healthcare Access and Quality (HAQ) Index

The HAQ Index is based on amenable mortality. Amenable mortality refers to the 32 causes of deaths that should not occur if healthcare were affordable, accessible, and effective. A sampling of these 32 causes ranges from vaccine preventable diseases, such as measles; infectious diseases, such as tuberculosis; chronic diseases, such as some cancers, stroke, and diabetes; gastrointestinal problems that surgery can cure, such as appendicitis; and maternal and neonatal disorders.

The HAQ Index is scaled from 0 to 100, with 0 the worst and 100 the best. Briefly, the HAQ Index is a measure of deaths that could be prevented by timely personal access to affordable, effective healthcare. Like the burden of disease, the Index allows for comparisons of amenable mortality across countries, between different populations, and over time.

In a nine-country peer comparison, the U.S. ranks last with a score of 88.7; Netherlands is best at 96.1, and the peer average is 93.7.[19] Not only do people living in Netherlands, Australia, Sweden, Japan, Austria, Germany, France, and the United Kingdom have *universal* access to effective care, but their healthcare systems are ranked in the top ninetieth percentile. In contrast, the American system is ranked in the eightieth percentile.

Although there is much debate regarding the relative contributions of behavioral factors, which include smoking, substance abuse, diet, and exercise; environmental factors; and socioeconomic factors, which include education and economic status, and so forth—HAQ data are risk standardized. Risk standardization eliminates behavioral and environmental factors that affect health and are outside the healthcare system's control; thus, risk standardization provides comparable measures of access to healthcare and its quality over time and place.

Despite the popular American myth that anyone can go to the local emergency department and receive all the healthcare they need, they cannot. By law, emergency departments are required to *stabilize* the patient—hence the phrase, "treat and street." Emergency departments do not provide prenatal care, teach diabetics how to adjust their insulin, nor work-up someone with a probable cancer diagnosis. Patients who need more than stabilization are referred to their primary care physician, which not all patients have, often because of cost. In contrast, top ranking countries have universal access to healthcare and limit their citizens' annual out-of-pocket costs. Not having health insurance is a huge barrier to access in the U.S. Ironically, even high-income U.S. adults report cost as a factor for avoiding healthcare; whereas, cost is not a limiting factor for low-income people in peer countries.

It's safe to assume one of the reasons for the U.S.'s low HAQ Index is due to personal lack of health insurance and unaffordable out-of-pocket costs. Evidence and precedent repeatedly show that working-age uninsured people are "more likely to receive too little medical care and receive it too late; be sicker and die sooner; and receive poorer care when they are in the hospital, even for acute situations like a motor vehicle crash."[20] Even people with insurance who have unpaid medical bills are less likely to seek needed care or fill a prescription.[21] Additionally, physicians can refuse to treat patients with outstanding medical bills and hospitals and surgery centers can require patients to pay for a procedure in advance, as long as it is not an emergency. However, of the insured, those with Medicaid suffer the most. A 2023 KFF report showed "Medicaid patients are more likely to report having problems finding providers who will accept Medicaid payment, experiencing denied or delayed approval for treatment, services, tests, and drugs; and that their insurance problems caused a decline in their health."[22]

## Hospital-Related Care

According to the 2021, KFF comparison data, the U.S. has more hospital admissions for asthma, diabetes, and congestive heart failure than peer countries. These admissions could be avoided with adequate primary care. The U.S. also performs more C-sections than peer countries, 317 per 1,000 births compared to the peer average of 256 per 1,000 live births. Although C-sections can be life-saving, they also have risks to the mother and the baby, and with the exception of Canada, the U.S. has more obstetric trauma during vaginal delivery, especially when instruments are involved. With the exception of Australia, the U.S. has more post-operative complications following hip and knee replacement surgery. Finally, the KFF comparison data show the U.S. has slightly higher rates of reportable medication, lab, and treatment errors than the average of its peers, 12.6% compared to 11.4%, respectively.[23]

On a positive note, according to the CF's comparison data for 2021, the U.S. compares favorably with ten peer countries for preventive care and patient engagement. Along with the United Kingdom and Sweden, the U.S. scored high on preventive care, such as mammograms and influenza vaccines. The U.S. and Germany scored highest on patient engagement, referring to patients and providers working together to discuss goals, priorities, and treatment options to improve health.

Unfortunately, due to frequent network changes by insurers, U.S. adults have the lowest rates of continuity of care with the same doctor.[24]

## Cost-Benefit Analysis and Policy Indications

Compared to similar wealthy countries, the international data show a large gap between the cost of healthcare and its benefit to Americans. Despite lower spending, peer countries have better health outcomes than the U.S., with its $4.5-trillion dollar healthcare system. At its average $12,914 per person cost, it's fair to say that Americans are not getting their money's worth.

Paradoxically, the high cost of U.S. healthcare contributes to poor health outcomes. For example, the maternal mortality rate in the U.S. is exceptionally high at 17.4 deaths per 100,000 live births, which is twice that of France, with next highest rate, of 7.6 deaths per 100,000 live births.[25] That 36% of all counties in the U.S. are maternity deserts—without obstetric services—is one contributing factor. On the other hand, considering that the U.S. system is for-profit, maternity deserts make financial sense, because maternity care is costly to provide and poorly reimbursed, with Medicaid covering about 42% of all U.S. births.[26] In contrast, top performing countries ensure continuity of maternity care, a longer length of postpartum care, and paid maternity leave.

The HAQ Index is another example of costs as a contributor to poor health outcomes. Peer countries have better amenable death scores for two reasons. First, healthcare is affordable: providing universal coverage and greater protection against out-of-pocket costs, peer countries have removed financial barriers to access. Second, peer countries invest in primary care that is conveniently accessible; do a better job of care coordination; and ensure that necessary services are geographically distributed to match the community's needs, thus, reducing geographic, economic, and racial discrimination. In contrast, the U.S. invests in specialty care; locates services where they are the most profitable; and struggles with care coordination because of reimbursement issues and physician turnover due to changing insurance networks.

## The High Costs of Low-Quality Healthcare

Just as a car in poor repair is more costly to operate than a car in good repair, an ineffective healthcare system is excessively costly to the nation. For individuals and families, the costs of healthcare's ineffectiveness are high in terms of lives lost, lost economic productivity, bankruptcies, and family disruption. For society, ineffectiveness increases the burden of disease, which costs more to treat than to prevent and is detrimental to national security.

According to a 2022 study by Deloitte,[27] untreated health problems associated with chronic diseases account for $320 billion annually, which if unaddressed could reach as high as $1 trillion by 2040. The $320 billion is a lot of unnecessary healthcare spending. To address these problems requires better prevention, earlier detection, timely interventions, better care coordination, as well as affordable and convenient access to care.

### Why the U.S. Has Poorer Health Outcomes than Peer Countries

Remember, all systems are perfectly designed to get the results they get. The international comparison data have been known by researchers and policy analysts—although not the general public—for decades. Why, then, is the U.S. healthcare system less effective than its peers? In systems language, why does the U.S. healthcare system produce poorer health outcomes than peer systems? The answers are found in Figure 5.1.

From a structural perspective, *access* to healthcare—hospitals, physicians, medical services, and prescription drugs—is of primary importance. Without access, people don't receive preventive care; chronic diseases go undetected and unmanaged; and treatable problems deteriorate into life-threatening physical and economic disasters. Access leads to better care, less burden of disease, better health, and longer lives. Access to healthcare results in better health outcomes at lower costs. From a compassionate perspective, access to healthcare reduces human suffering.

The U.S. also has a maldistribution of resources problem. Except for safety net hospitals whose mission is to provide care for the poor, hospitals locate in areas that have a preponderance of well-insured patients. Another example is hospital services with thin or negative margins, such as obstetrics, emergency departments and cancer care, not being offered, despite the community's needs.

Just as a key opens a locked door, health insurance opens the door to healthcare. As the data in this chapter show, a primary reason peer countries have better health outcomes than the U.S. is because the peer countries have some form of universal healthcare; their form of health insurance gives everyone access at an affordable cost. Peer countries also cap out-of-pocket costs at an affordable level for everyone. In contrast, about 10% of the American public do not have health insurance, another 38% do not seek healthcare because they cannot afford the out-of-pocket costs, and a few can't find care because some providers won't accept their health insurance, especially if it's Medicaid. It's fair to say that affordability is a major structural barrier to accessing healthcare.

Medical debt is also a cause of poor health outcomes. Research shows that being sent to collections is associated with poorer physical and mental health status, more

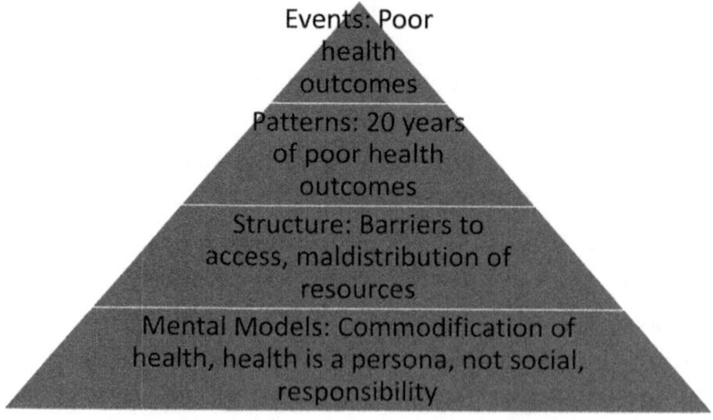


*Figure 5.1* The Iceberg Model of Systems

premature deaths, and higher mortality rates.[28] Not surprisingly, medical debt is concentrated among those least able to afford it. Whereas peer countries provide affordable care to everyone, American healthcare policies don't protect the working poor, the unemployed, and the uninsured from financial harm. Not surprisingly, the states with the highest levels of medical debt and its negative health consequences are those that didn't expand Medicaid. Despite federal policies requiring nonprofit hospitals to have financial assistance policies, the federal policies are seldom enforced and their requirements are so vague that too many patients fall through the cracks.

While insurance opens the door, access also refers to the availability of needed services, especially obstetrical services and primary care. Without the right resources in the right place, health insurance by itself cannot produce good outcomes. For starters, peer countries invest heavily in primary care, because, as its name suggests, *primary* care is the source of almost all preventive care, early diagnosis of treatable problems, management of chronic disease, and coordination of care among multiple specialties.

In contrast, the U.S. invests heavily in specialty care and under invests in primary care. For instance, the U.S. pay its primary care physicians significantly less than it pays its specialists. Moreover, both care coordination and chronic disease management are time consuming but insurers do not routinely pay well for either. As a result, care coordination and disease management are left to the patient as DIY, or do it yourself, the result of which contribute to the U.S.'s poorer health outcomes. Finally, peer countries do a better job of ensuring that necessary primary care services are geographically distributed to match the community's needs.

Ironically, healthcare's ineffectiveness is directly related to its inefficiencies. Systems thinking posits that a system is best understood by virtue of the behavior of the complex, interdependent *relationships* among its parts. Because the U.S. healthcare system is a for-profit system, the incentive is to maximize wealth, not health outcomes. Consequently, resources are distributed to profitable people, profitable service lines, and profitable geographic areas. With the ascendency of the financialization of healthcare, profits, which once were plowed back into the hospital to update facilities, modernize technology, and expand services, now leave the community and benefit investors.

## Mental Models Generate Structure

Mental models are the prevailing social values and beliefs that inform the structure of the U.S. healthcare system. Therefore, it's important to understand the values and beliefs that inform the U.S. structure, which, by design, limits access. Generally speaking, access to healthcare depends on how a country answers the question, "Is healthcare a public good or a consumer good"?

Long ago, other wealthy countries decided that healthcare is a public good. These countries value health as a social and economic asset—hence, universal access. They understand prevention and early detection help people be more productive throughout their lives and be more actively engaged in family and community activities. These countries understand that good prenatal and infant care pay off in the long run. Evidence and precedence show that healthy infants are more likely to have fewer health issues as adults; they are able to do better in school, have more stable relationships, and become more productive adults. These countries also understand that prevention and early detection cost less than intensive care after the disease has reached a crisis. In short, these countries value good health for everyone for economic, national security, and humane reasons.

In contrast, the U.S. has decided that healthcare is a private commodity—like a truck or a restaurant meal—accessible to those who can afford the purchase price. For those who can't, there's Medicaid if they meet stringent state requirements. Federally Qualified Health Care Clinics and safety net hospitals provide access, in some communities. For others, healthcare is given as a charity through free clinics and hospital charity programs.

Contributing to the commodity belief is a definition of health: the ability to work.[29] Which is one reason why in the U.S., health insurance is tied to employment and why some states with expanded Medicaid made working a prerequisite for Medicaid eligibility. Sadly, the U.S. is willfully blind to the fact that my neighbor's health affects my health. For instance, if my neighbor has a contagious disease, I might get it. If he has a poorly managed chronic disease, which causes him to often miss work, then I'm burdened with additional work and the concomitant physical and emotional stress. If his child is stressed in utero, which compromises adult productivity, then my taxes pay for the future welfare.

The effectiveness of any healthcare system is measured by how well it produces its product—health. Using health outcomes as a measure, the U.S. healthcare system is not nearly as effective as those of peer countries. Effectiveness is also a function of clarity of purpose. As a result of Americans having never clearly decided whether healthcare is a social good or a consumer product, the U.S. system is ineffective: It is fragment; access is a function of affordability, and resources are generally distributed by profitability rather than by need.

## Questions for the Reader

The questions provide an opportunity to examine your own mental models and values and to imagine other stakeholders' beliefs, fears, and values.

1 Are healthy citizens the backbone of national security and economic productivity? Why do you believe this; what might others believe?
2 What is your definition of health? Would your definition change if you had a chronic disease, suddenly disabled, or had a life-threatening illness?
3 What is the value to *you* of having good health yourself? To your family? Do you believe that your neighbors' and coworkers' health effects your health? Why do you believe this; what might others believe?
4 Should *everyone* in the U.S. have affordable health insurance, including the frail, disabled, elderly, those with part-time jobs, those with low-wage jobs, and gig workers? Why; what might others believe?
5 Were you surprised that the health outcomes produced by the U.S. healthcare system are not as good as its peers? If yes, what was surprising?

6 Do you, or anyone you know, live where maternity care is unavailable?
7 Do you, or anyone you know, live where the type of healthcare services you or others need is not available or not affordable? If so, what services are needed?
8 Do you know anyone who died younger than expected from a disease that could have been treated had it been diagnosed sooner? If so, how did that make you feel?
9 Do you, or someone you know, have a chronic disease? How well do you think it's managed? Do you have the information and resources you need to feel well most of the time? If not, what resources or help, if any, would be beneficial?
10 Do you know someone who died prematurely because they couldn't afford healthcare? What effect did the death have on the family? How did the premature death make you feel?
11 Do you, or someone you know, have multiple doctors caring for you? Who coordinates care for you? What resources or help, if any, would be beneficial?

## Notes

1 Brown, E.R. (1979). *Rockefeller Medicine Men: Medicine and Capitalism in America.* Berkley: University of California Press. p. 122.
2 Institute of Medicine (US) Committee on Quality of Health Care in America. (2000). Kohn, L.T., Corrigan, J.M., & Donaldson, M.S. (Eds). *To Err Is Human: Building a Safer Health System*. Washington, DC: National Academies Press (US). Available from: https://www.ncbi.nlm.nih.gov/books/NBK225179.
3 Johns Hopkins Medicine. (2016, May 3). Study Suggestions Medical Errors Are the Third Leading Cause of Death. https://www.hopkinsmedicine.org/news/media/.
4 Institute of Medicine (US) Committee on Quality of Health Care in America. *Crossing the Quality Chasm: A New Health System for the 21st Century*. (2001). Washington, DC: National Academies Press.
5 Institute of Medicine (US) Committee on Quality of Health Care in America. *Crossing the Quality Chasm: A New Health System for the 21st Century*. (2001). Washington, DC: National Academies Press. Executive Summary.
6 National Healthcare Quality and Disparities Report Chart Book on Patient Safety. (2023, March 22). *AHRQ Publication No. 23-0032 Updates 21–0012*. Rockville, MD: Agency for Healthcare Quality and Research. AHRQ Pub. No. 23-0032. PSNet. https://psnet.ahrq.gov/issue/national-healthcare.
7 Patient Safety Leader Reflects on 'To Error Is Human' Report. (2019, November 13). Podcast. https://www.aha.org/advancing-health-podcast/2019.
8 Schneider, E.C., Shah S., Doty M., et al. (2021, August). Mirror, Mirror 2021—Reflecting Poorly: Health Care in the US Compared to Other High-Income Countries. *The Commonwealth Fund*. https://www.commonwealthfund.org/press-release/.
9 Telesford, I., Wager, E., Amin, K., & Cox, C. (2023, October 23). How does the quality of the US health system compare to other countries. *Peterson-KFF Health System Tracker*. https://www.healthsystemtracker.org/chart.
10 Life Expectancy in the U.S. Dropped for the Second Year in a Row in 2021. (2022, December 22). https://www.cdc.gov/nchs/pressroom/nchs_press_releases/2022/20220831.htm.
11 Onque, R. (2022, August 29). Hawaii tops list of the 10 U.S. states where residents can expect to live the longest. *CNBC*. www.cnbc.com/2022/08/29/new-cnbc-report-hawaii-has-the-highest-life-expectancy.
12 Organization for Economic Cooperation and Development. (2021). [pdf] Health at a Glance 2021: OECD Indicators Highlights for the United States. *OECD*. http://www.oecd.org/unitedstates/health-at-a-glance-US-EN.pdf.

13 National Research Council (US); Institute of Medicine (US); Woolf, S.H., Aron, L. (Eds). (2013) *U.S. Health in International Perspective: Shorter Lives, Poorer Health*. Washington, DC: National Academies Press. Available from: https://www.nap.nationalacademies.org/catalog/1.

14 Emanuel, E., Gudbranson, E., & Van Parys, J. (2020, December 28). Comparing health outcomes of privileged US citizens with those of average residents of other wealthy countries. *JAMA International Medicine*. https://jamanetwork.com/journals/jamainternational.

15 Macrotrends. US Infant Mortality Rate 1950–2023. https://www.macrotrends.net/countries/USA/united-states/infant-mortality-rate. Accessed December 22, 2023.

16 Hassanien, N. (2021, December 22). Health of Black, Native moms key in fight to improve infant death disparities, experts say. *USA Today*. https://www.usatoday.com/story/news/health/2021/12.

17 Hassanien, N. (2021, December 22). Health of Black, Native moms key in fight to improve infant death disparities, experts say. *USA Today*. https://www.usatoday.com/story/news/health/2021/12.

18 Telesford, I., Wager, E., Krutika, A., & Cox, C. (2023, October 23). How does the quality of the US health system compare to other countries. *Peterson-KFF Health System Tracker*. https://www.healthsystemtracker.org.chart.

19 Telesford, I., Wager, E., Krutika, A., & Cox, C. (2023, October 23). How does the quality of the US health system compare to other countries. *Peterson-KFF Health System Tracker*. https://www.healthsystemtracker.org.chart.

20 Institute of Medicine (US) Committee on the Consequences of Uninsurance. (2002). *Care without Coverage: Too Little, Too Late*. Washington, DC: National Academies Press.

21 Plax, K., & Siefert, R. (2006). *Medical debt, healthcare access, and professional responsibility*. https://journalofethics.ama-assn.org/article/.

22 Diana, A., Rudowitz, R., & Tolbert, J. (2023, November 27). A look at navigating the health care system: Medicaid consumer perspectives. *KFF*. https://www.kff.org/medicaid/issue-brief/a-look-at.

23 Teleford, I., Wager, E., Amin, K., & Cox, C. (2023, October 23). How does the quality of the US health system compare to other countries. *Peterson-KFF Health System Tracker*. https://www.healthsystemtracker.org/chart-collection/quality-u-s-health.

24 Schneider, E. Shah, A., Doty, M., Tikkanen, R., Fields, K., & Williams, R. (2021, August). Mirror, Mirror 2021: Reflecting Poorly. Healthcare in the US Compared to Other High-Income Countries. *Commonwealth Fund Reports*. https://www.commonwealthfund.org/default.

25 Schneider, E. Shah, A., Doty, M., Tikkanen, R., Fields, K., & Williams, R. (2021, August). Mirror, Mirror 2021: Reflecting Poorly. Healthcare in the US Compared to Other High-Income Countries. *Commonwealth Fund Reports*. https://www.commonwealthfund.org/default.

26 Taylor, J., & Bernstein, A. (2021, August 10). The Medicaid coverage gap and maternal and reproductive health equity. *The Century Foundation*. https://tcf.org/content/commentary/medicaid.

27 Bhatt, J., Gerhardt, W., Davis, A., & Batra, N. (2022, June 22*)*. US health care can't afford health inequities. *Deloitte Insights*. https://deloitte.com/ng/en/our-thinking.

28 Han, X., Hu, X., & Zing, Z. (2024, March 4) Associations of Medical Debt with Health Status: Premature Death and Mortality in the US. *JAMA Network*. https://jamanetwork.com/journals/jamanetworkopen/.

29 Brown, E.R. (1979) *Rockefeller Medicine Men: Medicine and Capitalism in America*. Berkeley, CA: University of California Press. p. 122.

# 6 The U.S. Healthcare System Is Out of Date

## Effectiveness Means to Fulfill Its Purpose

Systems are a collection of parts, held together by networks of relationships, and organized to fulfill a purpose. The purpose of a healthcare system is to produce health. Effectiveness refers to the degree a system achieves its product, which, in this case, is health. As we've seen, the effectiveness of the U.S. healthcare system, according to a wide variety of health outcome measurements, compares poorly to other wealthy countries. Although there are multiple reasons why our healthcare system is not effective, three stand out.

The first reason is the lack of a clear purpose. Is the system to produce health or wealth? As a corollary, the U.S. doesn't have a clear purpose regarding whom healthcare is for. In contrast to other wealthy countries that give everyone access to affordable care, the U.S. distributes its resources to people, diseases, and geographic regions that are the most profitable, not the most in need of care.

Because the structure of a system determines its behavior, a second reason is its fractured structure. Unlike peer countries, healthcare in the U.S. is not *one* system but a mix of separate public and private providers and public and private insurers that are not integrated into one, universal system. Instead, these parts are organized to economically compete with each other to protect their own bottom lines. These baked in fracture lines compromise the system's ability to be effective at producing health.

The third reason is the structure of a system can become obsolete or fail to adapt to advances in either knowledge, technology, or significant changes in the types of disease. The controversial British epidemiologist, Thomas McKeown, was the first to show that types of sickness follow historical periods. Diseases of deficiencies—diseases of parasites and malnutrition—are endemic to hunter-gatherers infectious diseases are associated with widespread migration and rapid population growth; chronic diseases are associated with health-damaging societal factors and environmental toxins, seemingly endemic in postindustrial life.

Adaptation means changing the system's structure so the right parts and right relationships are organized in the right way so the system stays effective in a dynamic, changing world. The U.S. structure of healthcare system emerged during the time of acute, episodic diseases—such as infections and trauma, problems that

DOI: 10.4324/9781003538226-7

occur suddenly, last a short time, and health is restored. Therefore, it's useful to examine how the structure of the U.S. healthcare system has adapted as the types of diseases have changed over time and the understanding of their causes has evolved.

## The Biomedical Model of Disease

Figure 6.1 shows the biomedical model of disease, which is the core structure of the U.S. healthcare system. The content of its four core parts hasn't changed since the system was organized in the early 1900s. Based on the science and technology of the time, the BIOMEDICAL MODEL was "cutting edge" in the early 1900s. Then, the mind was separate from the body and disease was defined as a physical phenomenon, caused by one specific vector—germs, toxins, or trauma. Treatment was drugs and surgery. Licensed physicians were the sanctioned healer, socially responsibly for producing health. And, health was defined as the absence of disease.

A hundred and twenty years ago, medical care was in its infancy. Then the average life expectancy was 47 years. About 0.6% to 0.9% of women died as a result of childbirth and about 20% of children died before their fifth birthday. Trauma and infectious diseases were the major causes of death. Care was acute and episodic—broken bones were splinted, and wounds were kept as clean as possible. Chronic diseases were very rare since people didn't live long enough to develop them. Mental disorders were poorly understood and the responsibility of public health or the courts.

Since the 1950s, significant advances in science and technology have given people longer and more comfortable lives. However, today, chronic diseases have replaced acute infectious diseases as the leading cause of death and morbidity. Chronic diseases are largely preventable and caused by a multiplicity of factors. While lifestyle factors are the most often mentioned cause, chronic diseases are also strongly associated with unsafe environments and stressful social conditions. The point is the BIOMEDICAL MODEL, the core structure of the U.S. healthcare system, hasn't adapted to today's chronic diseases.

## The Biopsychosocial Model of Illness

The BIOPSYCHOSOCIAL MODEL of illness (Figure 6.2) was proposed in 1977, by George Engel, M.D., an American psychiatrist and pathologist. Based on his work with patients suffering from ulcerative colitis, depression, and pain, Engel's model is adaptive, including and going beyond the contents of the BIOMEDICAL MODEL in two important ways.

| **Cause** | **Treatment** |
|---|---|
| Biological pathology | Drugs & surgery |
| **Patient** | **Healer** |
| Person with biological pathology | Licensed physician |

*Figure 6.1* Biomedical Model of Disease

| **Cause** | **Treatment** |
|---|---|
| Biological pathology<br>*Psycho-social vectors* | Drugs & surgery<br>*Psychosocial support* |
| **Patient** | **Healer** |
| Person with pathology | Licensed physician |

*Figure 6.2* Biopsychosocial Model

First, Engel's model expands the pathological model of disease by positing that the *cause* of disease is multi-factorial, going beyond biomedicine's single-vector theory. Engel showed that psychological factors—in this case, coping skills and thoughts and feelings about one's self and the disease—and social factors—the patient's peer and family relationships, education, and socioeconomic status—were as important to the patient's vulnerability to disease, the severity of disease, and the response to treatment, as was the patient's biology.

Since 1977, Engel's studies have been further refined by other researchers. Scientific research in the areas of immunology, neurology, and endocrinology have proven the tight connections among biology, psychology, and social factors in the production of health and the cause of disease. Some examples of these tight connections are well known, such as the fact that people who are stressed are more susceptible to the common cold. Wounds heal faster for people in loving relationships. Other examples are less well known, such as people who are stressed—that is lack psychological resiliency and/or social and economic stability—are more susceptible to heart attacks, obesity, and autoimmune diseases, to name a few. Similarly, considered equivalent to smoking 15 cigarettes a day, people who are socially isolated and lonely have more health risks and shorter lives.

Decades of research have shown that stressful psychosocial factors are major factors in the cause and progression of chronic diseases. Simply speaking, stress is to the body as is driving a car that is low on oil, everything wears out sooner. Stress, whether it originates in psychological or social factors, can damage the body, as well as impede healing.

Similarly, decades of research have shown the tight relationship between psychosocial factors and *treatment*, the second adaption, or expansion, to the BIOMEDICAL MODEL. This adaption is especially important in the era of chronic diseases. For instance, people with heart disease who did not have someone to confide in were three times more likely to die early from their disease than those who were married or had a close friend. Diabetic patients who have positive feelings about their ability to cope with and manage their disease have better outcomes and are less likely to be depressed about their illness. Finally, multiple studies have shown that emotional well-being is strongly associated with lower mortality rates in people with chronic diseases.

Biomedicine eventually included psychosocial factors as part of its treatment, under the rubric of whole-person care. Referred to as patient-centered care, medical care expanded its clinical gaze. Doing more than treating the patient's pathology, patient-centered care refers to a large spectrum of patient needs, including his personality, emotional reserves, health literacy, family circumstances, and social needs. Patient-centered care respects the patient's choices, making him an active partner in the therapeutic relationship. It also refers to the time intensive coordination of the various medical and social services involved in caring for the patient.

Since 2001, patient-centered care is one of the National Academy of Medicine's six dimensions of quality. Safety, timeliness, efficiency, effectiveness, and equity are the other five. In organizations where patient-centered care has been well implemented, research shows that patient-centered care is associated with a higher rate of patient satisfaction with their physician, better adherence to prescribed treatment, better health outcomes, and more cost-effective care.[1]

## The Social Determinants of Health Model

The concept of social determinants of health (SDOH) is as old as Hippocrates, who posited health arises from a complex web of harmonious interactions among the individual and his social and natural environments. Over the centuries, the concept has fallen in and out of fashion, depending on conditions at the time. Based on an enormous amount of contemporary data showing the strong, reciprocal relationship between a country's economic growth and the physical health of its citizens, the World Health Organization, in the early 2000s, helped to reintroduce these concepts and their effects on health outcomes and health equity.

The Centers for Disease Control and Prevention (CDC) defines the SDOH as the conditions in which people are born, grow, work, live, and age, and the wider set of forces and systems shaping the conditions of daily life.[2] As discussed in the next sections, SDOH are upstream factors, such as public policy, cultural values, environmental conditions, social status, economic security, and lifestyle factors, to name a few, that affect health in positive and negative ways.

The SDOH posits that health is determined by the context of a person's life. SDOH are analogous to the nutrients in garden soil. Just as plants can't thrive in poor soil, neither can humans. Urban blight, violent neighborhoods, food deserts, run down schools, toxic waste dumps, lack of public transportation, and being homeless are some examples of "poor soil."

Just as plants thrive when the soil is rich but fail when the soil is poor, so does human health. Infamously known as the zip code effect, which means a person's zip code is a strong predictor of his health and longevity, the kinds of diseases he's likely to have, and his health outcomes. For instance, the largest gap in longevity in the U.S. is found in Chicago—a thirty-year difference between residents living on the wealthier north side from those living on the poorer, racially segregated south, nine miles away. Where one lives, one's zip code, determines not just access to healthcare but access to good education, good jobs, and a clean, safe environment, as well as overall quality of life—all of which affect health.

Poignantly, contemporary data show the societal conditions children experience in utero and during early childhood have a life-long effect. These early conditions influence learning abilities and behaviors, which, in turn, influences future earning

| **Cause** | **Treatment** |
|---|---|
| Upstream factors associated with biological pathology<br>*Public policy, cultural values, social status, economic and environmental conditions, lifestyle habits* | *Economic and social policies that improve economic and social status*<br>*Clean, safe environment*<br>*Lifestyle improvement* |
| **Patient** | **Healer** |
| *Population groups* | *Political and private entities, social institutions, including education and healthcare* |

*Figure 6.3* Social Determinants of Health Model

abilities. Early conditions also affect the size and strength of the future adult and establish much of the risk for chronic disease in adult life.

By acknowledging the upstream causes of disease, The SOCIAL DETERMINANTS OF HEALTH MODEL (Figure 6.3) presents a contemporary and radically different perspective from the BIOMEDICAL MODEL. In this model, the healthcare system is one of many social systems important to health. In this model, the patient is not an individual but a population, because, to use the cliché, one's health is generally the same as others living in the same zip code. Therefore, treatment includes but expands beyond drugs and surgery to include the more influential social, economic, and environmental policies that affect health, as well as a more equitable distribution of healthcare's resources. Indisputably it's better to prevent cholera by providing everyone potable water than to treat its victims, one-at-a-time with rehydration solutions and antibiotics. Or, to use the words of Archbishop Desmond Tutu, "There comes a point where we need to stop *just* (italics added) pulling people out of the river. We need to go upstream and find out why they are falling in." Two of the significant features of the SDOH model are (1) it identifies upstream causes prior to the presence of biological pathology and (2) indicates that other entities have more influence over the production of health than does medical care, i.e. the healthcare system.

Historically, attempts to improve health in the U.S. have been aimed at improving the quality and safety of medical care, that is, to make the healthcare system more effective. Since the 2000s, there's been increased recognition, however, that medical care contributes 10% to 20% to health outcomes. Genetics contributes another 5% and lifestyle factors contribute about 20%. The remaining 55% to 65% come from socioeconomic and environmental conditions.[3] Similarly, explaining the differences in mortality rates among the various regions in the U.S., especially the higher rate in the deep South, Healthy Democracy Healthy People, a coalition of national public health agencies, divided the relative contributions to health outcomes this way:

> We don't have these differences in health outcomes because of individual behaviors, it's related to the policy environments people are living in. … Your health is only 10 percent influenced by the medical environment and maybe 20 or 30 percent in behavioral choices. The social and political determinants of health are overwhelmingly what you're seeing in these maps.[4]

**WHO Schematic of the Social Determinants of Health**

The WHO conceptual framework (Figure 6.4)[5] presents a broader, deeper, and more complete understanding of health. First, it shows the causal and circular relationships among the wider set of forces and systems that impact health and well-being. Second, the arrangement of the categories from left to right shows a cascading effect, that is, each subsequent category in the causal chain of determinants is affected by the previous categories. The cascade starts with the Socioeconomic & Political context. Representing governmental, economic, social policies, and cultural values, this structural category is the most influential and the most resistant to change. Structural refers to macro-level laws and policies supported by long-standing cultural and societal values. Structural determinants are so embedded in daily life they are usually invisible and taken for granted, making them difficult to change.

At the end of the cascade are the Intermediary Determinants—Material Circumstances, Psychosocial Factors, Behavioral Factors, Biological Factors, and the Health Care System. Intermediary determinants refer to tangible factors, such as lifestyle choices, adequate housing and food, and social support. They are tied to one's social position. Healthcare's placement as an intermediary determinant indicates the structure of the healthcare system, distribution of its resources, and health outcomes are strongly influenced by the structural determinants.

Third, the multi-directionality of the arrows shows that the production of health is dynamic and multi-factorial. Significantly, the multi-directionality of the arrows shows the reciprocity between health, social position, and the country's economic and social policies, and its cultural values. The reciprocal link between economic

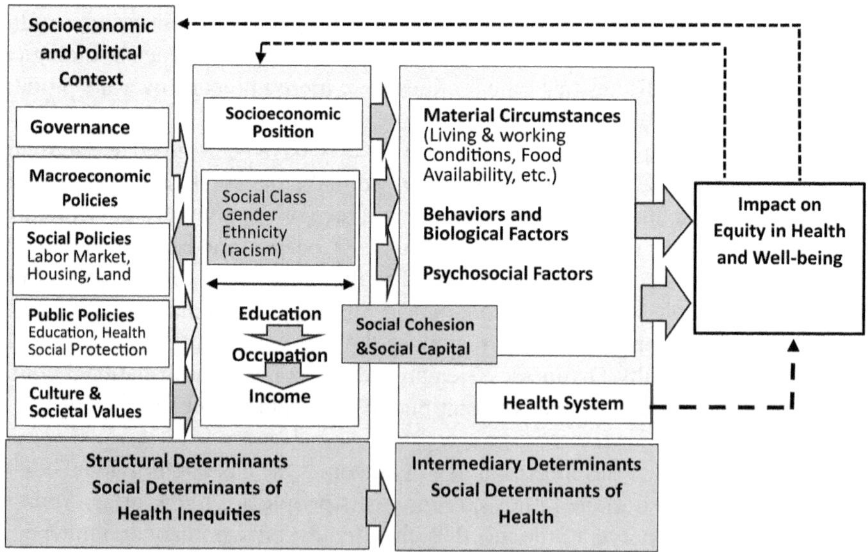


*Figure 6.4* WHO Social Determinants of Health

and political conditions and physical health has been understood since the early Industrial Revolution. Both Edwin Chadwick, a British bureaucrat and social reformer, and Rudolph Virchow, M.D., a German pathologist, polymath, and social reformer, pushed for social and political reform, convinced that ameliorating wretched living and working conditions would do more to improve health than biomedicine could ever do by treating the sick one at a time. Both understood that poverty and pollution were not just vectors for personal illness but that personal illness and political stability are intertwined and the absence of either is costly to the economic and social stability of a country.

Finally, the circularity of the arrows between health equity and well-being (health) and the structural determinants forms a cycle, which is mostly unacknowledged in the U.S. The multi-directionality of the arrows shows that health (well-being) and health equity feed back to the structural determinants. Cycles repeat themselves … unless they are disrupted. Which is why the health of grandchildren tends to be the same as the grandparents.

**Where's the Leverage?**

The schematic of the WHO SDOH is like the Iceberg Model of systems thinking. Both help distinguish events, or what is easily visible, from their root causes, or the wider set of forces and systems that affect health. Typically, we focus our attention and efforts at the events level—reducing costs for some, increasing access for others, adding more quality measures here, taking away services there. Yet, healthcare's costs continue to rise and health outcomes continue to fall, despite our best efforts.

The strength of the WHO schematic is it reveals the upstream forces—the social, political, and economic systems—that dictate the structure of the U.S. healthcare system and affect health outcomes. The downside of the schematic is because the pathway between SDOH(s) and disease is not always straightforward, but long and complex, often dependent on the length of exposure, the toxic load, and the presence of other variables, these upstream causes are often denied or disputed. For example, the tobacco industry was able to deny, for years, that smoking causes cancer. The effect of climate change and gun violence on health are two more emotionally charged examples.

Just as mental models are to understanding and leveraging healthcare's structure, the WHO schematic also reveals a deeper level of understanding of upstream political, economic, and other forces that determine health outcomes. This deeper level of insight reveals the greatest leverage for improving health outcomes is at the policy level. In contrast to the BIOMEDICAL MODEL, which improves the health of one person at a time, policy changes improve the health of whole populations at a time. A famous example is John Snow, M.D., prevented the spread of cholera in a poor area of London by removing the handle of the water pump serving the area. Another example is the Medicare legislation, which gave 19 million Americans health insurance in 1965. Today, about 66 million Americans are enrolled in Medicare. Because of the potential effect of policy to improve health outcomes, policy should be investigated when considering the root causes of health outcomes.

### Socioeconomic and Political Context

Operating through laws, social policies, and cultural values, the influence of the Socioeconomic & Political category is formidable. On one hand, rooted in this category are the laws, social policies, and cultural values that determine the allocation of public and private resources to healthcare, that, in turn, determines the effectiveness, efficiency, and equity of the U.S. healthcare system. Within this category are economic policies that make the U.S. system for-profit; that make insurance coverage disease-specific; tie health insurance to employment; and variegate reimbursement by private and public payers, as well as geography. Within this context are policies that determine why not everyone has access; why working White men are more likely to have health insurance than working men of color; why providers are paid less for caring for Medicaid than Medicare patients; and why most providers prefer to care for those with private insurance.

Here, too, are court decisions that overturned Roe vs Wade, a decision that took decisions about women's reproductive health away from the patients and into the hands of the states. Here, too, are cultural values that champion the self over the community; stigmatize certain diseases, like HIV, mental illness, and obesity; stigmatize the poor and People of Color; and promote the belief that access to care is not a human right but something people earn.

Also, within the Socioeconomic & Political category are the laws, social policies, and cultural values that are distinct from the healthcare system but are powerful determinants of health, such as those affecting the quality of the environment. Just as plants can't be healthier than the soil in which they grow, a healthy environment is vital to human health. While a healthy environment is free of air pollution, toxic chemicals, contaminated water, and violence, equally important a healthy environment also contains safe neighborhoods, nearby grocery stores, good schools, healthcare, recreation, and transportation.

Complex social programs also originate in the Socioeconomic & Political category. While the entire set is important, food security and housing stability are absolutely critical to good health. The Supplemental Nutrition Assistant Program, or SNAP, commonly known as food stamps, which helps about 13% of the U.S. population, is critical to the development of healthy minds and bodies of children. Despite the assistance, about 22% of Black households, 21% Hispanic, and 9% of White households don't have enough money for food, according to U.S. Department of Agriculture data.[6] Despite the importance of food to young minds and bodies, in 2024, fourteen Republican-led states turned down a summer federal program that provides food aid to low-income children. While costly to low-income families, the communities lost the multiplier effect a few more dollars would have had on the local economy.

Similarly, housing instability is an ongoing issue with about 37.1 million families affected according to Healthy People – 2030, despite multiple federal government programs to help with this issue.[7] Housing instability is associated with poorer health, a 5–9 times greater chance of dying prematurely, a greater risk of mental illness, as well as negatively affecting the physical, emotional, and mental development of children.

Biomedicine's narrow perspective—that health is an individual concern and curing disease is the responsibility of licensed physicians—ignores the many ways in which the Socioeconomic & Political structural determinants not only determine the design of the U.S. healthcare system, but affect health outcomes. Although the category's influence tends to be overlooked, a close examination of this mostly invisible category reveals how the U.S. answers three questions: "What health burdens matter"? "Whose burdens matter"? and "Who's responsible for producing health"?

## Socioeconomic Position

The second structural category, the Socioeconomic position, refers to a population's position, or status, in the general society. A population is defined as a group of people who share similar characteristics, such as health conditions, like asthma or pregnancy; demographic features, like age, gender, race and ethnicity; geographic features like zip code, rural, and urban; and socioeconomic status, like income, education, and occupation. Depending on their circumstances, people can be part of multiple populations at the same time. Black pregnant women with Medicaid insurance and inner-city children with asthma are two examples of people being part of multiple populations.

Populations are ranked as high or low status, or somewhere in between, according to a combination of their education, occupation, income, gender, and ethnicity/race. As underscored by the study showing a thirty-year gap in longevity between populations living in Chicago's highest and a lowest-income zip codes, decades of robust evidence show a direct correlation between socioeconomic position and health. Like being at the top of a ladder, those ranked higher live longer and have less burden of disease than those in the socioeconomic strata below them. The Socioeconomic position is a structural category because gender and ethnicity/race are fixed and social mobility (typically, a function of education and occupation) tends to be more fixed than fluid in the U.S., compared with peer countries.

Socioeconomic position, or ranking, is a determinant of health because it determines a population's access to social assets. Socioeconomic position determines the amount of agency, or control, people have over their lives; the kinds of choices they can make; the kinds of community resources that are available; and how easily they can access the community's resources. Socioeconomic position determines a population's ability to earn a living; live in a clean, safe environment; afford housing and transportation; and have access to healthcare, healthy food, and a good education, as well as having leisure time and access to recreation. Also, socioeconomic position influences the right to live with dignity and respect. The amount of existential stress a person experiences is in direct relationship to his socioeconomic position.

The multi-directional arrows between Socioeconomic Position and Socioeconomic & Political categories indicate reciprocal influence. The arrows represent the concepts of social cohesion and social capital, which will be discussed in Chapter 8. Briefly, the more social capital a population has the more it can influence laws and social policies in self-favorable ways.

The effect of socioeconomic position on health was definitively proven by the landmark Whitehall study. The ten-year study, which began in 1967, compared the mortality of men working in the highly stratified British civil service and showed that the men in the lowest status jobs were three times more likely to die prematurely than men in the highest status jobs. The men in low status also had a greater prevalence of cardiovascular morbidity, which was attributed to their higher incidence of smoking.

Twenty years later, the study was repeated. Known as Whitehall II, the second study included woman and cancer, lung disease, depression, etc., as well as cardiovascular disease. Briefly, the study showed that "the way work is organized, the work climate, social influences outside work, influences from early life, in addition to health behaviors … contributed to the social gradient in health … lead[ing] to the uncomfortable (for some) finding that inequalities in health cannot be divorced from inequalities in society."[8]

At the root of the high maternal death rate for Black women are structural racism and sexism. Black women are two to four times more likely to die from pregnancy and childbirth than White women, regardless of education and socioeconomic status. For instance, Beyonce and Serena Williams—two world-famous, privileged Black women with access to healthcare—almost died giving birth. Indisputably, access to resources and variation in quality of care are contributing factors, the overarching explanation for the higher incident of maternal deaths for Black women is the term "weathering." Coined by Dr. Arline Geronimus, weathering refers to the premature biological aging and associated health risks caused by the stress of racism and social adversity.

The loss of social position is associated with deaths of despair. Coined by Princeton economists Anne Case and Angus Deaton, deaths of despair are deaths from drug overdoses, suicide, and alcoholic liver disease. Since the early 2000s, deaths from these causes have risen so greatly that they are considered as a major contributor to the drop in U.S. life expectancy. While their incidence varies by age, geographic region, education and ethnicity, deaths of despair disproportionately affect White, working-class males who've experienced economic hardship and a loss of social status.

The common denominator to these various studies associating lower social position with poorer health status is stress. Stress is defined as the demands of a situation are greater than one's resources to meet or mitigate the demands. Briefly, chronic stress keeps the body's "fight, flight, freeze, and faint" responses turned on. Like being perpetually chased by the proverbial tiger, the constant, low-grade release of cortisol and other stress hormones eventually harms the body's immune, endocrine, and nervous systems, leading to downstream pathology. Like an engine running too hot—whether referred to as chronic stress, or weathering—the damage is inevitable and irreparable.

### Inter-Dependent Relationship Between Socioeconomic Position and Socioeconomic & Political Context

The COVID-19 pandemic highlighted the health inequities associated with social inequities. In response, Centers for Medicare and Medicaid Services (CMS), along with The Joint Commission and other national organizations, established new quality measures to promote health equity. Most of the measures require screening patients for "health-related social needs (HRSN)," such as food security, housing stability, transportation, and so forth. The intent is for hospitals to partner with community organizations to provide one patient-at-a-time with the resources they need to be healthy.

Although the mandate is well-meaning, it assumes the community resources are readily available and are easy to qualify for, which is not the case. Most community social services are already tapped out, are difficult to qualify for, and have long wait lists. Implicitly, this mandate makes health providers responsible for solving social inequities while letting upstream policymakers off the hook. Politicians and judges, not physicians and hospital administrators, legislate the broader, structural social policies, their funding, and establish the rules that are either inclusive or exclusive.

Generally speaking, people who live on the East and West coast live longer than people who live in Appalachia and the Deep South, and White live longer than Black people. However, White Americans don't live as long as their counterparts in Canada and Western Europe. When asked why, given the legacy of White privilege, three sociologists from the University of Cincinnati opined "Whiteness encourages whites to reject policies designed to help the poor and reduce inequality because of animosity toward people of color as well as being unaware that the poor include a great many white people."[9]

### Intermediary Determinants

The SOCIOECONOMIC POSITION sets the stage for the INTERMEDIARY DETERMINANTS. These are material circumstances, psychosocial circumstances, biological factors, and the health system itself. Behavioral factors are often included in this category. As their name indicates, these factors are *intermediary*; they are the link between SOCIOECONOMIC POSITION and HEALTH. As intermediary factors, there's an assumption of personal choice. There's the common belief that low status people choose to engage in risky behaviors—eating high-fat diets, smoking, abusing drugs, etc.—that result in poor health. However, choice is a function of agency and not everyone has enough social status to choose. Given the disparity in social position, those at the bottom of the social ladder have fewer choices and less autonomy.

Despite the prevailing stereotypes of race and poverty, most people at the low end of the wage scale work hard. Most people who seek care at free clinics or *Federally Qualified Health Centers*—federally funded, walk-in clinics that offer care on a sliding fee—have at least one job and often several. They would make the right choices—if they could. The higher incidences of cancer, heart disease, diabetes, obesity, and substance abuse are found among the more vulnerable members of society because they *are* more vulnerable. Given the disparity in income, they have less agency. Agency, to a great extent, is bestowed by the laws, social policies, and cultural values that determine who is in and benefits and who is out and loses.

Material circumstances refer to things like housing stability, food security, clean, safe neighborhoods, and access to education, grocery stores, and healthcare. Material circumstances also refer to the built environment, such as roads, sidewalks, water and sewage systems, transportation, community gardens, safe parks and places to recreate, as well as the geophysical environment, or clean water, air, and soil. Like well-amended garden soil, the better one's material circumstances the better one's health.

Psychosocial factors include being appreciated and respected for one's work and other social contributions; having positive family relationships; having a network of supportive and trustworthy friends and associates; being included in social and professional groups; and having good personal coping skills, optimism, and a sense that one's life matters to others. Psychosocial factors are protective for they indicate that one belongs, is respected and held in esteem, and has some agency, or control over one's life, all of which signify safety. Safety, which is an antidote to stress, includes but is more than physical safety. Safety also includes social stability without which leads to feelings of anxiety, dissatisfaction, and disaffection, which over time damage delicate neuroendocrine, immunological and other biological mechanisms, resulting in "weathering," or observable, deleterious changes to the brain and body, with physical disease and poor mental health being the end result.

Biological factors refer to age, gender, and genetics, which, although they belong to the individual, are outside the individual's control. In contrast, behavioral factors, also known as lifestyle factors, the individual has some control over, at least in theory. Behavioral factors include a healthy diet, frequent exercise, enough sleep, the avoidance of tobacco, alcohol, and illicit substances, and having a circle of friends. Poor lifestyle habits are commonly associated with chronic diseases. For instance, smoking is associated with many kinds of cancer; obesity is associated with diabetes, heart disease, high blood pressure and some cancers; and alcohol is associated with chronic heart disease, liver diseases, high blood pressure, and some cancers. Finally, diseases of despair—alcohol abuse, drug overdose, and suicide—have behavioral and psychosocial, as well as socioeconomic antecedents.

Because chronic diseases are associated with behavioral factors, and because biomedicine historically places the locus of health on the individual patient—not the population—interventions are typically aimed at the patient, specifically exhortations to develop better lifestyle habits. The problem is lifestyle habits are notoriously difficult to change. Although it's well known that social policies that affect behavior are more effective—for example mass public campaigns and raising taxes on tobacco products have done more for smoking cessation than individualized interventions—it's easier to blame the victim. There's the prevailing belief that poor lifestyle habits are a function of personal failure—not enough will power to make good choices or a lack of discipline to work hard enough to be successful.

In some cases, personal failure is true. There are patients who are unwilling to help themselves, and there are some who resist lifestyle changes, knowing there's a pill to lower cholesterol, a nicotine patch to stop smoking, bariatric surgery and Ozempic to reverse obesity, and so forth. And, there are some who are willing and able to change. However, these changes come more easily to people who have adequate material resources and social support than to those who live in socially adverse conditions.

For others, the opportunities for healthy habits lie outside their control. For instance, doctors often tell diabetic and overweight patients "to eat more fruits and vegetables." While valid, the exhortation eclipses other realities, such as 17% of

Americans are low income and live in food deserts.[10] For them, their social position and material circumstance precludes access to healthy foods. Instead, they depend on food banks and convenience foods where fresh meats, fruits, and vegetables are not always available.

In 2021, 32.1% of all U.S. households below the federal poverty line were food insecure, compared with about 12% of all US households.[11] Around 30 million students qualify for free or reduced-price school lunches and about 450,000 children participate in the "Backpack" program, receiving non-perishable food to carry them through the weekend. Food is one of the basic human needs, and the link between poverty and obesity is strong. Unfortunately, many nutritional needs could be mitigated by better public policy—raising the federal poverty level so more people are eligible for food stamps (SNAP); raising the SNAP average per person allowance from $4 dollars per day to the real cost of a day's worth of food; lowering the cost of healthy foods—fresh fruits, vegetables, and meat; and raising the costs of empty calorie, convenience foods, which are titrated with the trifecta of salt, sugar, and fat that is associated with obesity.[12]

The healthcare system is an intermediary determinant because of its intersectionality between the personal aspects of health and healthcare delivery. Because of its intersectionality, the healthcare system has a strong advocacy role, according to the WHO. The WHO posits that the healthcare system can improve equitable access to effective care; influence upstream, structural governmental and economic policies that affect health, access to healthcare, and distribution of healthcare resources; and advocate for the vulnerable, assisting them in the acquisition of needed material and social resources, such as food, shelter, transportation, and job accommodations for people with disabilities. Ideally, those inside healthcare, who have the knowledge and experience, are the best advocates. However, historical evidence indicates, the capacity of the U.S. healthcare system to affect the structural determinants of health is inherently limited.

Finally, the circularity of the arrows between health equity and well-being (health) and the structural determinants of health forms a cycle, which is generally unacknowledged. The cycle is important, however. First, it shows the tight connections between structural determinants of health and health. Like the chicken and the egg, the cycle shows that poverty creates poor health and poor health creates poverty. For example, children living in households without enough food, have trouble learning, don't go to college, get low wage jobs, and the cycle repeats. Second, since the turning of the cycle has either a positive or negative effect on future generations, the schematic shows until the cycle is broken children who grow up poor today are likely to have poor health as adults and be the parents of tomorrow's poor children who will also have poor health, *ad finitum*.

## Population Health Management

Population health management (PHM) offers a new discipline within the healthcare industry. This discipline is based on the Tripple Aim, proposed in 2007 by the Institute of Healthcare Improvement (IHI). The IHI is an internationally recognized leader in improving health outcomes and healthcare systems across the world. According to the IHI, improving the U.S. healthcare system required the simultaneous pursuit of three aims: Improve health of *select* populations, improve the patient's experience, and reduce the per capita costs of care.

PHM extends care beyond the traditional dyad of physicians and hospitals, requiring partnerships with other community organizations, such as public health departments and social service organizations. It also expands the care team beyond the physician to include non-physician providers, nurses, pharmacists, social workers, and others.

As a discipline within the healthcare industry, PHM modernizes and reorganizes the delivery of care to fit with today's prevalence of chronic diseases. Chronic diseases, such as cancer, heart disease, diabetes, etc., are the leading cause of death and disability in the U.S. Chronic diseases account for 90% of today's healthcare costs, as well as contributing to lost wages and lower productivity.[13]

The purpose of PHM is to manage the health outcomes and costs of care for a *select* population. Select refers to a defined patient population under the care of a physician or set of physicians; select doesn't include everyone in the community or zip code. Populations can be selected according to any number of criteria, ranging from geography of the service area, ethnicity, insurance carrier, or diagnosis, or a combination of any of these or other criteria. Once selected, the population is further stratified by risk, including age, history of use of expensive services, number of chronic diseases, mental health or substance abuse issues, and social position. Care is coordinated and targeted to the population's needs. Periodically, outcomes are reported to ensure quality and accountability.

Costs are controlled in several ways. The first is to keep healthy people healthy, through regular check-ups and preventive care—vaccinations and routine screenings, such as mammograms and blood pressure checks. Another is to treat complex and catastrophic illnesses at centers of excellence, which have the resources and experience that small, local hospitals rarely have.

Costs are also controlled by managing chronic diseases to prevent complications and hospitalizations. Care management involves the physician who guides the coordination of care and is supported by a team of health professionals. This involves both coordinating the care the patient is receiving from multiple physicians so that nothing gets dropped or overlooked and controlling costs by eliminating redundant and low-value tests and procedures. Care management also includes actively engaging the patient in his own care.

Finally, care management includes identifying and attempting to ameliorate unfavorable *intermediary*, not structural, SDOH that lead to poor health outcomes within the population. While this requires addressing lifestyle habits, such as smoking and food habits associated with obesity, it more recently includes monitoring for housing instability, food insecurity, access to transportation, feeling safe at home, and the ability to pay utility bills. This amelioration of *Intermediary Determinants* is typically done through community partnerships, although some large hospital systems use their own resources. For instance, Boston Medical Center has a rooftop vegetable garden to provide fresh vegetables to food insecure patients.

Los Angeles county is planning to convert a mostly vacant hospital into affordable housing units. The Henry Ford hospital in Detroit created a laundry business in a low-income area that pays $15 per hour. And, Northwell Health in New York City has implemented prenatal and postpartum services across the city to reduce maternal mortality and pregnancy-related health risks in Black women. While these hospitals are some of the leaders in PHM, not all hospitals have the resources and not all communities have or can afford such community resources, unfortunately. Although valuable to those who are included in the *select* population, intervening one-patient-at-a time at the intermediary determinants level maintains the status quo. By focusing on intermediary determinants, Population Health Management (PMH) eclipses the effect laws and policies have on the health of everyone living in the zip code, for instance.

The third aim—reduce the per capita costs of care—opened the door to moving away from traditional fee-for-service to value-based reimbursement. With fee-for-service, hospitals, doctors, and others are paid by "volume," which means each provider is paid a fee for each service provided. The more volume, the more income. With value-based care, services are bundled, and physicians and others are paid based on meeting specific health outcomes and cost-efficiency benchmarks. Hence the adage, "no outcome, no income." Although value-based reimbursement helps insurers control their costs, it puts doctors and hospitals at financial risk, something small, independent hospitals may not be able to afford. It's yet to be seen the extent these cost-savings are passed on to patients through lower insurance premiums.

In this era of chronic diseases and health disparities, PHM offers a proactive way to focus on health and disease prevention in select populations through financially linked providers and community partnerships. One of the most well-known PHM pioneers is Kaiser Permanente. Through their focus on preventive care and community partnerships, they are providing better health outcomes, more health equity, and better cost management. Kaiser Permanente is successful because clinical care and health insurance are part of the same, vertically integrated system. This eliminates any incentive for either the insurance arm or the clinical arm to take financial advantage of the other.

How quickly or widely PHM will be widely adopted is unclear. Three large barriers block easy adoption. One barrier is the cost of analytical software. PHM is data driven, but the software is enormously expensive and is rapidly changing, and generally unaffordable for many small hospitals and physician groups. A second significant barrier is community partnerships. Small communities may not have the necessary social services—such as mental health, housing and food assistance, and so forth—needed to ameliorate the intermediary SDOH. Large communities may have the resources but are often already at maximum capacity. The third large barrier is reimbursement. Because value-based reimbursement requires physicians and hospitals to assume some of the risk, both have real financial concerns about switching from fee-for-service to value-based reimbursement, especially if their service area is rural or small where there are no economies of scale, or they are an urban safety-net hospital.

## PHM Is Not the Same as the Social Model of Health

The American Hospital Association (AHA) defines PHM as "the process of improving clinical health outcomes of a defined group of individuals through *improved care coordination and patient engagement* (italics added) supported by appropriate financial and care models."[14] While there's no doubt that PHM is a good fit for managing chronic diseases and reducing some health disparities, it's unrealistic to expect PHM to raise the health status of Americans to the level experienced by other wealthy countries. While effective for producing better health outcomes for defined groups of individuals, PMH is a variation of the BIOMEDICAL MODEL. It treats individuals, one-at-a-time. PHM tacitly maintains biomedicine's out of date pathological model of disease. It also maintains the notion that good health is simply a personal concern—a commodity for those who can afford it. It does not make healthcare more affordable for anyone. PHM continues to fragment care instead of providing universal access to healthcare and, finally, focuses on the intermediary determinants of health and ignoring the structural SDOH, PHM is a low leverage intervention. With hospitals accepting responsible for improving health, PMH conceals the role of laws and policies in determining health and maintains the belief that drugs, surgery, and a healthy lifestyle are the primary producers of good health.

The SOCIAL MODEL OF HEALTH, however, shows the production of health is complex. The social model goes beyond the biomedical concept that health is a personal commodity. The social model posits that humans literally embody the very fabric of their society. Good health involves more than biological factors. Human life is one of the most tightly coupled systems in the universe. Humans are linked to the external world through the five senses. Our eyes, ears, nose, mouth, and skin are portals, so to speak, bringing the external environment into the physical self. The material world is incorporated into the physical body through the food, water, and air we imbibe. Likewise, social and personal encounters enter our bodies through our eyes, ears, and skin, affecting effect our nervous, endocrine, and immune systems, which signal inclusion and safety or exclusion and danger. Good health is dependent upon the upstream cultural values and political policies, which affect midstream the social and geophysical environments in which people live, work, play, and age, which finally affect one's physiology. Because higher status people have the benefit of a richer social fabric, they tend to live longer and have less burden of disease than lower status people.

In the support of equitable health outcomes, the Biden administration, in 2023, published *The US Playbook to Address Social Determinants of Health.*[15] The three pillars of the Playbook encourage (1) public private partnerships to work together to improve data gathering and analytics, (2) to use funding from a variety of sources, and (3) to increase the number of and strengthen "backbone" organizations, or organizations with the capacity to coordinate and manage community-based care. While a step in the right direction and acknowledging that solutions must include upstream economic and environmental factors, the Playbook recommendations are piecemeal, local community interventions. These interventions do not address upstream political and economic policy that are at the root of the U.S.'s poor health outcomes.

## Systems Thinking Redux

The Iceberg Model (Figure 6.5) is a reminder that all systems are perfectly designed to get the results they get. Chapter 5 showed the effects of limited access and maldistribution of resources on health outcomes. This chapter shows the effect of the SDOH—especially the two structural SDOH—on health outcomes. It also shows that these determinants are not distributed equitably throughout the U.S. and that 80% of them are beyond healthcare's control. The chapter indicates that the healthcare system has reached the edge of its capacity to produce health. While this doesn't mean that drugs and surgery are ineffective—they are effective—it does mean that to treat someone with drugs and surgery and return them to the "poor soil" of their social status and expect them to become healthy is unrealistic.

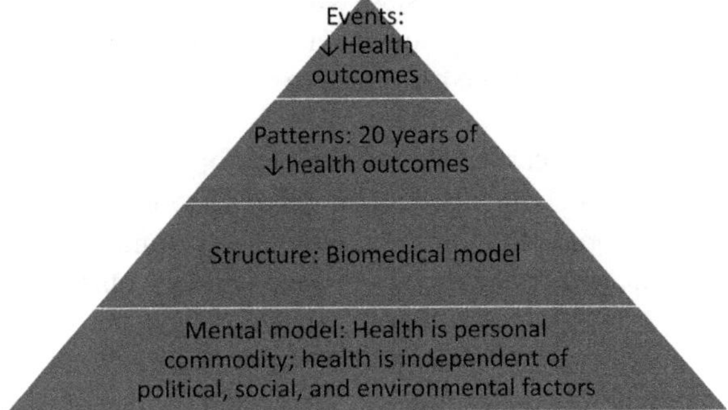


*Figure 6.5* Iceberg Model: A 20-Year Effect of the Biomedical Model on Health Outcomes

Importantly, this chapter indicates that the healthcare system, a vitally important system, is one social system among many that determines health. As a corollary, this chapter shows there are limits to the healthcare system's effectiveness and that to expect better health outcomes requires public and private attention to the two structural SDOH. For these upstream issues, which originate outside the healthcare system's boundaries, it seems that the best role of those inside the healthcare system is advocacy for healthier social and economic policies and a more affordable, inclusive system.

## Questions for the Reader

The questions provide an opportunity to examine your own mental models and values and to imagine other stakeholders' beliefs, fears, and values.

1 Is good health a personal responsibility, only? Why do you believe this; what might others believe?
2 Go to the website County Health Rankings National Findings Report.[16] Click on "Explore Health Rankings," click on "Find Data By Location" and enter your zip code. How does the health ranking of your county compare with your state and national rankings?

3 Are good health habits important to health? How would you rate your health habits? What might you need to have a healthier lifestyle?
4 Is living in an area that has clean air, water, and soil important to health? Is your environment free of toxins and pollutants? Should all citizens live in a healthy environment? Who is responsible for a clean, safe environment: healthcare, the government, corporations, others? Why do you believe this; what might others believe?
5 Does a person's social position and/or race contribute to their health habits and/or their health status? Why; what might others believe?
6 What should the role of your doctor and/or hospital be to assure you are food secure, have stable housing and transportation, and are able to pay your utility bills? Why; what might others believe?
7 For people who don't have the basics, who should they turn to for help? Their family, their church, community social services, the federal government? Does your community have adequate resources to help everyone in need? Why; what might others believe?
8 Who is responsible for caring for vulnerable populations, e.g. the poor, frail elderly and disabled, people who live in dangerous or toxic environments, the marginalize, and People of Color? The federal government, state governments, cities, the churches, non-profit social services, families, other? Why; what might others believe?
9 The U.S. healthcare system represents 17.3% of the U.S. GDP, are you in favor of the U.S. spending less on healthcare and more on other social programs, such as education, housing, childcare, for example. Why; what might others believe?

## Notes

1 Gluyas, H. (2015, June 13). Patient-centered care: improving healthcare outcomes. *Nursing Standard.* https://journals.rcni.com/nursing-standard/patient.
2 CDC. (2022, December 8). Social Determinants of Health at CDC. https://www.cdc.gov/about/sdoh.
3 Distribution of Determinants of Health *Source:* Tarlow, A.R., & St. Peter, R.F. (2000) (Eds). *The society and Population Reader: A State and Community Perspective* (Vol. 2). New York: New Press. pp. x-xi.
4 Woodard, Colin. (2023, September 1). America's Surprising Partisan Divide on Life Expectancy. *Politico.* https://www.political.com/news/magazine/2023/09/01/.
5 World Health Organization. (2010, July 13). A Conceptual Framework for Action on the Social Determinants of Health, Discussion Paper 2. *WHO.* https://www.who.int/publications/i/item/9782941500852.
6 Bleich, S.N., Koma, J.W., & Jernigan, V.B.B. (2023, November 30). The worsening problem of food Insecurity. *JAMA Health Forum.* https://jamanetwork.com/journals/jama-health-forum/fullarticle/2812589.
7 Healthy People – 2030. *Housing Instability.* https://health.gov/.../housing-instability.
8 Ferrie, J.E. (Ed). (2004). Work, Stress, and Health: The Whitehall II Study. *WorkStress.net.* https://workstress.net/sites/default/files/whitehall_11_study.pdf.
9 Woodard, Colin. (2023, September 1). America's Surprising Partisan Divide on Life Expectancy. *Politico.* https://www.political.com/news/magazine/2023/09/01/.
10 Which cities have the most people living in food deserts? (2021, June 23). *USA Facts.* https://usafacts.org/articles/which-cities-have-the-most-people-living-in-food-deserts.

11 USDA ERS Food Insecurity and Nutrition Assistance. (2023, November 29). https://www.ers.usda.gov/.../food-security-and-nutritional-assistance.
12 Pollan, M. (2006). *The Omnivores Dilemma: A Natural History of Four Meals*. New York: Penguin Press.
13 The cost of chronic disease. (2022, February 10). *BCBS Progress Health*. https://www.bcbsprogresshealth.com/data/the-cost-of-chronic-conditions.
14 AHA. Population Health Management. https://www.aha.org/center/population-health-management.
15 Domestic Policy Council Office of Science and Technology Council (2023, November). The US Playbook to Address Social Determinants of Health. https://www.whitehouse.gov/...11/SDOH-Playbook-3.pdf.
16 2022 County health ranking national findings report. *County Health Rankings & Roadmaps*. https://www.countyhealthrankings.org/reports/2022.

# 7 Health Equity

## Why Health Inequity Is Important

Healthy people are the backbone of a productive country. They are the brains and brawn of a strong economy and national security. The purpose of a healthcare system is to produce health, instead, the U.S. healthcare system is better at producing wealth than health. As previous chapters have shown, compared with peer countries, the U.S. healthcare system is less effective in producing health, despite spending almost twice as much as its peers. We've seen how the U.S. healthcare system falls short in three of the four hallmarks of a healthy system—efficiency, effectiveness, and production of the expected product. Equity, which is the fourth hallmark, also shows poor systemic performance.

Equity is not the same as equality. Equality means everyone gets the very same resource; whereas, equity means everyone gets the resource they need. Imagine three people of different heights trying to pick apples from a tree they need ladders to reach. Equality means that each gets the same size ladder, even though the ladder is not tall enough for the shortest person to reach the tree. In contrast, equity means that everyone gets the size of ladder he needs to reach the apples on the tree.

Equity refers to the fairness built into a social system. Simply speaking, fairness refers to who is included in the system and benefits and who is excluded and loses. Health equity is defined by the Centers for Disease Control and Prevention (CDC) as "the state in which everyone has a fair and just opportunity to attain their highest level of health." Using more poignant words, Joni Eareckson Tada puts it this way:" The hallmark of a healthy society has always been measured how it cares for the disadvantaged."[1]

Health equity is measured by health disparities. Health disparities refer to the differences in health outcomes between different populations. Originally defined by Healthy People 2020, health disparities refer to a particular type of health differences of populations of people "who have systematically experienced greater obstacles to health based on their racial or ethnic group; religion; socioeconomic status; gender; age; mental health; cognitive, sensory, or physical disability; sexual orientation or gender identity; geographic location; or other characteristics historically linked to discrimination or exclusion."[2] Measured in terms of health outcomes, such as longevity and burden of disease, health disparities are avoidable and unfair.

DOI: 10.4324/9781003538226-8

## The U.S. Healthcare System Is Designed to Be Unfair

To understand the unfairness baked into the structure of the U.S. healthcare system, a quick review is in order. In the early 1900s, when the structure was solidifying, medical doctors consolidated their power and privilege through scientific authority, educational credentialing, and the enactment of licensing laws. Hospitals began to be known as a place for curative medicine, shifting care of the sick from a woman's domestic chore to a professional responsibility. In the early 1900s, the healthcare system was split into two. One half belonged to the medical profession, known as private practice, which claimed for itself the treatment of sick individuals. The other half was assigned to public health, which was responsible for sanitation and bacteriology research. Care of the indigent and People of Color (POC) was also assigned to public health, which fit with racial and class biases at the time.

At the beginning, the delivery of care was separated into two systems: private medical care for those who could afford it and indigent care provided by the government. From the start, private medicine was opposed to any form of public or compulsory insurance, and any expansion of public facilities to provide non-indigent care.[3] However, private medicine did support the public investment of hospitals and graduate medical education.

## A Brief History of Political Attempts for Universal Access

By national policy the U.S. has piecemeal, not universal, access to healthcare. Universal access depends on some form of universal health insurance. Despite multiple attempts, the U.S. has not found the political will to provide Americans with universal access to healthcare. Universal access has been a political debate since 1915, when reformers issued the first major proposal for national health insurance. In 1945, President Truman proposed a national health insurance plan, which American would pay for with a combination of taxes and fees. In 1970, Senator Edward Kennedy introduced a bipartisan bill proposing universal health insurance to be financed by payroll taxes and general federal revenue. In 1993, President Clinton proposed a huge, sweeping, and complex plan to provide universal coverage. Clinton's plan, which was built on the existing mix of public/private insurance and the belief that market competition could control costs, was envisioned as a synthesis of liberal and conservative values. Like the Truman and Kennedy proposals, the Clinton plan was not enacted into law. Finally, in 2012, after much congregational wrangling, President Obama's Affordable Care Act was finally passed. Although more people had insurance coverage, coverage wasn't universal.

The same political and cultural forces that stopped the 1915 reform attempt—resistance from powerful interest groups who profit from the status quo, fear of socialized medicine and government control, fear of rationing, racism, beliefs that the free-market can control costs, and conservative values that healthcare is a commodity and a personal responsibility, not a social good—have endured for a very long time.[4] Instead of universal access Americans have piecemeal access to for-profit healthcare.

## Instead of Universal Access the U.S. Has Unequal Access

Access to healthcare is important to achieving health equity for all Americans. Briefly, access to care means having: (1) health insurance, (2) timely access to urgent care, (3) a usual source of care from a provider the patient has a relationship with, and (4) access to routine preventive, screening, disease management care, and rehabilitation care.

For starters, unlike peer countries, not everyone in the U.S. has health insurance. Without health insurance, access to healthcare is significantly compromised. Multiple studies have shown that working age Americans without health insurance tend to be sicker and die sooner. They receive too little medical care—they tend not to receive screening, prevention, or disease management services—and the care they receive is too late. For example, the uninsured are far more likely to undergo diabetic amputations and die much earlier from cancer due to too little care that's often too late. Finally, they receive poorer care when hospitalized, even for serious problems like motor vehicle accidents.[5,6]

For a variety of reasons, even with health insurance, Americans don't have equal access to healthcare. For instance, health insurance controls the network of physicians and hospitals patients have access to. Physicians and hospitals tend to locate in well-insured locations, often leaving poorer, inner-city and rural areas without access to either urgent or routine care. Finally, not all physicians and hospitals accept all health insurance. This is especially true for Medicaid, and, in some places, hospitals are not accepting some Medicare Advantage policies. Moreover, health insurance determines what benefits are covered, an issue that has become problematic, especially for patients who respond better to brand name than generic drugs or need a diagnostic test their insurer overrules.

Among its peers, the U.S. is the only country that ties health insurance to employment. This tie reinforces the definition of health—the ability to work—and the cultural belief that health benefits are earned as a moral reward for being productive. Tying health insurance to employment makes the employer the arbiter of the covered benefits. This may work for some families but not others, depending upon the family's health problems. Whereas peer countries provide all of their citizens with the same slate of covered benefits, the U.S. does not.

Because insurance companies offer a wide range of covered benefits at varying prices, what gets covered depends upon what the employer is willing to pay for. The employer is also the arbiter of the size of the network of hospitals and physicians, and the amount the employee pays for healthcare. Tying health insurance to employment also leaves employees at the mercy of their employer. Employees who are fired, laid off, or even lose their job because they are too sick to work lose their health insurance. On the other hand, health benefits can tie employees to jobs they'd like to leave, because to leave would be to lose their health insurance. Although most people who leave their jobs are eligible for COBRA insurance, many find they can't afford the premium. COBRA refers to the federal law, Consolidated Omnibus Budget Reconciliation Act of 1985, that allows eligible employees and their dependents to purchase their workplace insurance for a limited time.

About 55% of Americans have employer-subsidized health insurance; however, not *all* workers are covered. For instance, low-wage workers and their families are often without health insurance because they (1) aren't offered employer-subsidized insurance, (2) can't afford their share of the premium costs, or (3) earn too much to qualify for Medicaid but not enough to afford insurance through the Exchange. Because health insurance benefits are not taxed as income—for example an employer-paid health benefit worth $1,000 a month is $12,000 in income that is not taxed—the uninsured lose twice. Ironically, of the approximate 10% of Americans without health insurance, over half live in families with one or more full-time workers.

## Medicaid Magnifies Healthcare's Unfairness

Although Truman's attempt to provide universal insurance failed, by the time Lyndon Johnson was president two large groups of Americans were without health insurance: the elderly and the poor. Their inclusion came through Medicaid and Medicare, part of Johnson's Great Society legislation. Medicare, which is for seniors, is a national insurance program that is paid for by workers and employers through mandatory Federal Insurance Contributions Act (FICA) taxes. Medicaid is a public health insurance program paid for by a combination of federal and state funds. Like Truman, Johnson faced stiff opposition from special interest groups, who made it crystal clear that the legislation was not to make healthcare a right. Therefore, the laws and regulations made sure that Medicare and Medicaid conformed to the U.S.'s cultural and political values regarding race and class. Medicare was something seniors had earned through prior work, whereas, Medicaid was charity.

Medicaid is a public health insurance program for qualified, low-income people. In 2023, Medicaid is the largest health insurer in the U.S., covering about 95 million Americans, or about 27% of the adult population and about 50% of all children. Medicaid is a federal-state funded program, with each contributing about 50% of its costs. Because each state manages its own program, eligibility and covered benefits vary widely from state to state.

Conservatives often refer to Medicaid as a safety net program for the truly needy. However, Medicaid was never designed to function like private health insurance for low-income families, or cover all low-income people, or cover all illness, or cover all diagnostic tests and treatment. Instead, it was designed to cover certain low-income populations such as the blind, people with specific disabilities, and the elderly needing nursing home care. It was not designed to cover the working poor.

Knowing that many low-income people couldn't afford private health insurance but earned too much to qualify for Medicaid, the Affordable Care Act attempted to close the insurance gap by expanding Medicaid. For states that have chosen Medicaid expansion, coverage now includes families making less than 138% the federal poverty level. And, for the first time, coverage includes non-disabled adults without children. In contrast, in the ten states that have not expanded Medicaid, non-disabled adults are ineligible for Medicaid, regardless of how low their incomes.

Intermittently, Congress has expanded Medicaid's minimum eligibility requirements and increased its covered benefits, especially for children, people with disabilities, and pregnant women. In 2023, with the intent to reduce the U.S.'s high maternal death rate, and since Medicaid covers 40% of the pregnancies in the U.S., the Biden administration gave states the option of increasing post-delivery care from two months to twelve months. Thirty-six states took advantage of this option the first year it was enacted.

For states that expanded Medicaid, the documented benefits are impressive. On the health side of the ledger, expansion improves access to care and increases the use of preventive care, resulting in better chronic disease management, better health outcomes, better cancer survival, and less mortality. The narrowing of racial-related health disparities is also associated with these benefits. The benefits on the financial side of the ledger are equally impressive. For the patient, there's more financial stability, less food insecurity, fewer evictions, as well as more productivity. For hospitals, there's less uncompensated care and more financial support for rural and safety net hospitals. And, for the states, the federal government pays 90% of Medicaid costs, instead of the 50% that the unexpanded states receive. States have used these extra dollars to offset other healthcare costs.

**Physician Inequities**

Not only is the U.S. healthcare system designed to be unfair to the patients, but it's also deliberately designed to be unfair to its physicians. Prior to the early 1990s, physicians charged Centers for Medicare and Medicaid Services (CMS) for the services they provided according to what was considered customary and reasonable. Because some physicians pegged their charges much higher than others, there was considerable variance in what CMS paid. Looking for ways to improve payment uniformity, CMS outsourced payment decisions to the American Medical Association. Briefly, because specialists controlled the committee, the standardized physician fee schedule rewards specialists. This has resulted in a large and widening gap between the incomes of those who spend time with patients—primary care physicians, geriatricians, pediatricians, psychiatrists, and internists—and those who do procedures—cardiologists, surgeons, interventional radiologists, and other specialists.

Due to significant inequities in income, the U.S. has a shortage of and maldistribution of primary care doctors. They are the specialists who provide the preventive care and do the care coordination, resulting in better outcomes and lower healthcare costs. Although the solution is to change the fee schedule to incentivize primary care, there are multiple barriers that are unlikely to be overcome.

**De facto Rationing Contributes to Health Inequities**

All countries employ some form of rationing to control healthcare costs, although the methods vary. Peer countries ration care vis-à-vis a global budget, which is an explicit form of rationing. Global budgets are a commitment to economic efficiency and to a predetermined level of care for every citizen.

Most Americans believe that the U.S. healthcare system is free of rationing. In fact, fear of rationing is why many Americans are against universal healthcare. Special interest groups with large profit margins—such as big Pharma and the insurance industry—exploit the public's fears of losing benefits, losing the freedom to choose their own doctor, and longer wait times for medical appointments, diagnostic tests, and surgery. Instead of counteracting these misleading claims, neither the regular media nor the echo-chambered social media tell the public that citizens of other wealthy countries pay half what Americans pay for healthcare, that their wait times are similar to America's, and that their citizens live longer and are healthier than Americans.

The reality is that Americans experience extensive de facto rationing through the affordability of health insurance, out-of-pocket costs, the wide variation in covered benefits, and resources distributed according to profitability rather than need. Physician choice is limited due most insurer's narrow networks; post COVID-19 wait times have significantly increased for almost all specialties. Americans also experience other forms of de facto rationing by age, gender, race, and geographic location.

## Geographic Inequities

Geography is a form of de facto rationing, thus a source of health disparities. Health disparities are differences in the health status of a particular group when compared to the overall population of a country. Because the U.S. healthcare system is for-profit, it makes sense that healthcare's resources are not equitably distributed but are mostly found in the profitable geographic locations. While geographic access to healthcare's resources contributes to health disparities, disparities tend to be associated with other forms of rationing such as race, income, and age. This is a reason why high poverty regions, like Native American reservations, inner cities, and rural areas have a greater burden of disease and shorter longevity.

Small rural hospitals represent about 35% of all U.S. hospitals; however, for many reasons, many rural hospitals are financially insecure.[7] Rural residents tend to be older, have a greater burden of disease, and shorter life expectancy than urban residents. Since 2010, the life expectancy for rural Americans has slightly dropped (0.2 years for women and 0.3 for men) but has slightly increased for urban Americans (0.6 for women and 0.3 for men).[8] According to the National Rural Health Association, deaths from heart disease, cancer, and respiratory disease account for the greatest differences.

Different rural areas are burdened with different health problems. For instance, it's well known that the highest rates of death from heart disease are not randomly scattered throughout the U.S. but occur largely in one place known as the "Coronary Death Valley," an area that includes most of Appalachia, which is characterized by unemployment, isolation, and poor health habits. Similarly, a higher rate of stroke-related mortality is found in the "Stroke Belt." Located in the southeast U.S., it is characterized by higher concentrations of obesity, smoking, and high blood pressure, with Southern-born Blacks more at risk for high blood pressure than Blacks born elsewhere. Similarly, the maternal mortality rate is higher in rural areas than urban. Among the states, maternal mortality is highest in Tennessee, Kentucky, Alabama, and Arkansas, which also have high concentrations of maternity deserts, large populations of Black people, and structural racism.

The cause of these health inequities is inequitable distribution of resources. About 20% of the U.S. population lives in rural areas, but only 5% of physicians practice there. Compared to urban communities, rural communities have fewer doctors and hospitals. Rural residents also have less access to specialty care, preventive care and chronic disease management, and maternity services. Rural residents also have longer travel times. Rural communities are less likely to have employer-sponsored health insurance, and their poor are usually not poor enough to qualify for Medicaid. Besides barriers to access, rural residents are more likely to have poor lifestyle habits, more social isolation, more poverty, and higher rates of alcohol and substance abuse, all of which contribute to health disparities.

Prior to COVID-19 about 40% of rural hospitals had negative operating margins. During COVID-19, federal relief funds provided a financial lifeline. After COVID-19, federal relief funds ended but staffing shortages and inflation caused expenses to soar, leaving about 30% of rural hospitals at the risk of closure. Because hospital closure does multiple harm to rural communities, communities look for ways to protect their hospital. Being desperate, one enterprising community in rural Pennsylvania opened a GoFundMe campaign to raise $1.5 million needed to keep its doors open.

The fragility of rural hospitals can be traced to reimbursement policies, inequitable distribution of resources, and the cultural value that healthcare is a commodity, available to those who can afford the purchase price. Most rural hospitals lose money delivering care because reimbursement doesn't cover the cost of the delivery of care. Bluntly speaking, rural hospitals have too many Medicare and Medicaid patients and not enough privately insured patients. Whereas large hospitals use the better reimbursement and their large volume of privately insured patients to make up the inadequate Medicare and Medicaid reimbursement, rural hospitals don't have that option.[9] To add insult to injury, CMS frequently threatens to cut funding to its "Disproportionate Share Hospital" program, a program that helps safety net and rural hospitals offset the costs of uncompensated care.

Mortality rates tick up when a rural hospital closes.[10] To protect rural residents, the Consolidated Appropriations Act of 2021 established the Rural Emergency Hospital (REH), a new type of hospital. In exchange for a $3.2 million annual payment, rural hospitals will provide only outpatient and emergency care and close all inpatient services,[11] assuming that inpatient care will be provided at larger hospitals elsewhere.

Despite the financial incentive, the REH solution may only worsen health disparities. One is the ability to transfer patients. Since larger hospitals are struggling with their own staffing crisis, many are unwilling to accept transferred patients from hospitals that are not part of their own system. Bad weather and bad roads can make timely transfers difficult, a problem for critically ill patients or a woman having a baby. And, families of rural patients may not be able to afford the extra costs of travel, food, lodging, and time away from work. The are other downsides, too.

The reduction of care leaves the community with outpatient and emergency services, only. Slimmed-down healthcare is an impediment to recruiting new workers and new businesses to the community. Moreover, it's unclear whether the provision of prevention and chronic disease management services, important to the reduction of health disparities, will continue with REH hospitals.

### Economic Inequities

Historically, poverty in the U.S. is usually associated with rural communities and large urban centers. Poverty is a major cause of poor health. People living in poverty have a greater burden of disease, higher mortality, and shorter life expectancy. They are also at higher risk for mental illness. In the U.S., the largest group of poor are children.

Up to 60% of a population's health status is determined by its zip code. As has already been mentioned, Chicago, which has the greatest health disparities, the life expectancy between the wealthiest and poorest zip code varies by 30.1 years.[12] Zip code is shorthand for the kinds and quality of resources available within the postal area. Although access to healthcare is important, other factors are more important. There's little doubt the thirty-year gap between Chicago zip codes is due to the two structural social determinants of health (SDOH): SOCIOECONOMIC AND POLITICAL CONTEXT and SOCIOECONOMIC POSITION.

The protective and health producing benefits of possessing a high socioeconomic status, or being wealthy, are well known. Wealth provides material benefits, such as access to healthy foods, safe, clean neighborhoods, and good schools. Wealth gives people more choices and more autonomy, buffering them from a myriad of everyday stressors. Finally, more wealth means more political influence, which easily becomes a virtuous circle, each one increases the benefits of the other.

Volumes of evidence show that cities with the greatest gaps in life expectancy are those most segregated by race and ethnicity, compounded by poverty, high housing costs, and subpar social services.[13] Ineluctably, race, poverty, toxic environments, and lack of resources, like good schools, healthy food, and affordable healthcare, cause long-term suffering. Their negative effect on health is felt from infancy through adulthood. From childhood forward, poor living conditions increase the risk of autoimmune diseases and chronic diseases, such as diabetes, asthma, obesity, and shorten longevity.

To add insult to injury, decades of research show that the human nervous system interprets poor living conditions as not safe. This increases the likelihood of anxiety, depression, and other mental health issues in adults and children. Unfortunately, for children, the effect is lifelong. Growing up in unsafe, or stressful, conditions compromises their ability to learn, form meaningful relationships, and be healthy, productive adults. The most painful of all is that the neurophysiological—weathering—effects of this stress get passed on *in utero* from one generation to the next. Poverty is the gift that keeps on giving, from one generation to the next.

Despite the prevailing stereotypes of poverty, generally speaking, people are poor not because they don't work hard enough or make good choices; people are poor because they are the vulnerable members of society. Society's political and economic policies and its cultural values have determined who is in and benefits and who is out and loses.

## Racial Inequities

The CDC defines racism as "a [social] system of structures, policies, practices, and norms that assigns value and determines opportunities based on the way people look or the color of their skin. This results in conditions that unfairly advantage some and disadvantage others."[14] Compared to White people, the disadvantaged are the POC. Recognizing that people belonging to different races and ethnicities have preferences about the terms used to describe them and have their own unique experiences with healthcare, this degree of specificity is beyond the scope of this book, therefore, the term People of Color is used and inequities are generalized, unless otherwise noted.

In every state in the U.S., and by every metric, racial and ethnic minorities have poorer health, more preventable hospitalizations, and a greater burden of disease. Compared with Whites, POC also have a shorter life expectancy. For example, the life expectancy of Black people is an average four years shorter than White Americans. Similarly, more than twice the number of Black infants die before their first birthday than White infants and Black women are more likely to die following child birth than White women. Black patients are 42% more likely to die following surgery than Whites, and young Black males and teens are twenty times more likely to die from gun violence than their White counterparts.

The sources of racial disadvantages range from the structural—political and economic policies and cultural values—to the interpersonal, affecting all aspects of life. On one hand, structural racism minimizes society's investment in basic necessities for POC, such as access to affordable housing, healthcare, and education; good jobs; and clean, safe environments. For instance, in 2022, an average of 10% of Americans didn't have health insurance, or to drill down, 22% of Hispanics, 10% of Black, and 6% of White Americans were without health insurance, respectively.[15] Medicaid expansion lags behind in states where there are slightly more POC than White. Structural racism also contributes to the perennial withdrawal of federal and state dollars for food stamps, housing vouchers, and other supportive services that would advance health equity.

## Implicit Bias

Implicit bias also affects the kind of care POC receive and whether they seek care or not. Implicit bias refers to negative attitudes that healthcare workers have toward POC. Implicit bias can also refer to healthcare workers' biases about gender and age. In 2003, the National Institutes of Medicine (IOM) released the book, *Unequal Treatment: Confronting Racial and Ethnic Disparities in Health Care.*[16] The product of a national committee of experts, the landmark book confronted the painful truth that, even after accounting for socioeconomic factors and having health insurance, the quality of the medical care POC received was significantly affected by race and ethnicity.

Generally speaking, POC receive poorer treatment than White people. POC are less likely to receive relief for pain, less likely to receive stents for heart disease, and less likely to receive expensive care or necessary therapeutic drugs, even with insurance. Because of poor chronic disease management, they are more likely to need diabetes-related amputations. Because POC are less likely to receive adequate and other diagnostic tests, they are also less likely to receive an accurate diagnosis. The cost of racial and ethnic inequities is high, about $451 billion in 2018, primarily from expensive late-stage treatments, lost work productivity, and premature death.[17]

The most poignant revelation of the IOM study was that, despite structural factors that restrict access to resources and amplify the stressors of daily life for POC, the implicit bias—stereotyping and prejudice by care givers, even though largely unconscious—caused providers to misdiagnose and undertreat POC. Highlighting the effect of implicit bias, a 2023 study showed that in communities with more Black doctors, Black people lived longer.[18] Because only 6% of physicians,[19] 8% of nurses,[20] and 12% of hospital CEOs are Black,[21] the unequal care is found across all clinical settings—private and public hospitals, as well as teaching hospitals.

As a result of its finding, *Unequal Treatment* contained 21 recommendations to reduce inequities within healthcare itself. A short list of the recommendations includes increasing the number of minority doctors and nurses; more training about implicit bias, or diversity training; more patient navigators and community health workers; and more use of evidence-based care. The book also recommended equalizing access to better health insurance, instead of the cheaper, poorer coverage plans commonly used by POC.

Twenty years later, the National Academy of Medicine, the rebranded name of the IOM, convened another consensus committee to revisit the *Unequal Treatment* report. The Committee's purpose was to review progress since 2003 and examine the current state of racial and ethnic inequalities. The 2023 Committee discovered that racial inequities persist and the structural racism behind the inequities is seemingly intractable, a challenge made worse by the Supreme Court's 2022 ruling striking down affirmative action in higher education. Although some progress has been made, it's been uneven. There's still much work to be done and the lack of progress is expensive. As with the case in resolving complex systemic problems, there is a cascade of racial-related health inequities to be remedied, all of which is made more difficult by a fragmented healthcare system.

## Gender Inequities

Gender bias in healthcare is another cause of health inequity. Research and experience show that gender bias against women in healthcare is old, endemic, and contributes to poor health outcomes. Generally speaking, women tend to receive poorer care than men. For example, heart attacks in women are often misdiagnosed and fewer women than men receive coronary artery bypass surgery. Cancer is one of the leading causes of premature deaths in women that could be prevented by early detection and access to optimal care. Women are less likely than men to have their symptoms taken seriously; they are less likely to receive a timely diagnosis; they are more likely to be misdiagnosed or receive improper treatment; and they are less likely to receive Cardiopulmonary resuscitation (CPR) in public places. Their pain is more likely to be discounted or seen as "all in their heads." Drug side effects are more common in women than men, primarily because until the 1980s, new medicines and treatments were mostly tested on men. And, annually, women pay about 18% more for healthcare than men of the same age, even when pregnancy care is excluded.[22]

Some of the problems women encounter stem from medical researchers' use of the Reference *Man*, a statistically average size male with a standard set of biological and physiological parameters. Since the 1920s, Reference Man is the physiological model for diagnostic criteria, clinical trials, and medical research. Concomitantly, research into women's health issues has historically been underfunded. Although, starting in the 1980s, researchers began investigating the physiological differences between males and females, the differences between their physiology have yet to become the norm. Consequently, many doctors today still believe that female bodies are like male bodies. As a result, female symptoms that differ from typical male symptoms are likely to be overlooked or discounted, leading to delayed or wrong diagnosis and treatment. And, since drugs and their dosages continue to be based on the male body, women have a greater risk of side effects.

Despite the differences in physiology between men and women, gender bias against women is part of the American culture. Gender bias is also one of the structural SDOH. The bias is so common it's taken for granted. For instance, health providers tend to interrupt women more frequently than men, and women patients often feel they have not been heard—typical in regular society. Because of the bias, many women find that their health problems are not taken seriously; that their opinions about treatment options are not sought or are overridden; and that those who speak up and advocate for themselves get labeled as pushy and ungrateful. All of which leads to poorer care.

The structural gender bias is as old as the Comstock Act of 1873, which banned the mailing, distribution, and possession of information and devices related to abortion and contraception. (The act also included obscenity.) The Supreme Court's overturning of Roe vs Wade, the harsh penalties imposed by multiple states against anyone helping a woman get an abortion, and the Texas federal judge who suspending the FDA's twenty-year-old approval of Mifepristone, an abortion drug, reflect the structural gender bias that affects the delivery of healthcare to women and undermines women's rights to control their bodies and their health.

Women of color have a second strike against their health—racial discrimination, another structural SDOH. The intersection of race and gender is an unhealthy place to be. Statistically speaking, healthcare providers give lower priority to Black women and Black women are treated with less respect and receive lower quality of care. Also, Black women are 41% more likely to die of breast cancer, 60% are more likely to have high blood pressure, and more likely to experience intimate partner violence than white women.[23] Plus, the maternal mortality rate for Black women is almost three times greater than it is for White women. In short, Black women are disproportionately affected by health disparities, the majority of which arise from structural SDOH, or as Walton said, "Black women's biggest health issue is the system."[24]

Although the LGBTQ+ community includes men as well as women, health disparities among this variegated group are well documented and tied to discrimination and significant sexual and social stigma. Among this group, they have problems obtaining health insurance, are frequently homeless, and almost 30% reported providers wouldn't see them because of their gender identity.[25] And, their health outcomes are worse than their heterosexual peers. With the shortage of providers who understand the LGBTQ+ culture and their diverse health needs, the LGBTQ+ community struggles to receive compassionate care that meets their needs. Although the needs vary considerably among this variegated group, they include HIV, certain cancers, homelessness, substance abuse, depression, and gender dysmorphia, to name a few. Finally, transgender healthcare has been politicized, with several states enacting laws that ban transgender care.

## Mental Health Inequities

Mental health is a broad term that covers a range of mental, behavioral, addictive, social, and emotional issues. About 15 million Americans live with a serious mental illness. According to 2022 data from the National Alliance for Mental Illness, one in five adults experiences a mental illness, one in twenty adults experiences a serious mental illness, and one in six youth between the ages of six and seventeen experiences a mental health disorder each year. Fifty percent of life-time mental illness begins by age fourteen and 75% begins by age twenty-four, and suicide is the second leading cause of death in youths between the ages of ten to fourteen.[26]

Mental disorders cast a long shadow. Severe mental disorders can reduce life expectancy by ten to twenty-five years.[27] This is because about 65% of people with mental or substance abuse disorder also have at least one chronic disease, and about 25% to 35% of those with a chronic disease also have a mental disorder. Mental disorders are also the largest cause of years lived with disabilities, worldwide.[28] For people of any age, mental illness has a negative impact on all areas of their lives, including school and work performance, supportive relationships with family and friends, and participation in community and other social functions.

The COVID-19 pandemic had a widespread, negative impact on mental health. According to the U.S. Surgeon General, the pandemic exacerbated a pre-existing mental health crisis in children and teenagers. Unsurprisingly, the poor and POC suffered more. They entered the pandemic with poorer mental health and had fewer SDOH benefits to buffer the stressors of COVID-19, as well as having less access to mental health services than wealthier White citizens.

According to a 2022, Kaiser Family Foundation (KFF) report, 90% of adults surveyed believed that COVID-19 put the U.S. in the midst of a mental health crisis.[29] Numerous studies showed a record increase in deaths from drug overdose, a rise in suicide rates, and a 30% increase in teen age visits to emergency departments for mental health reasons. In short, the COVID-19 pandemic worsened long-standing mental health problems. Although COVID-19 exacerbated a mental health crisis, it did bring the inequitable care for mental disorder to the front and center of nation's awareness and exposed the web of inequities designed into the U.S. healthcare system regarding mental health care.

At the center of the web is Descartes' error—that the mind is separate from the body. This innocent error—the separation of the mind and body—was the prevailing scientific belief at the start of the 20th century, when the U.S. healthcare system was in its infancy. As a result, society gave the body to healthcare and the mind to the church and the law. At the beginning of the 20th century, healthcare's boundaries excluded the care of those with mental disorders.

Since World War II, tremendous advances in pharmacology and neuroscience have greatly improved some aspects of caring for people with mental health and substance abuse disorders. However, the vestiges of Descartes' error, such as the lack of national investment in either mental health facilities or practitioners and the fact there are twice as many mentally ill in U.S. prisons and jails than in treatment facilities, are readily apparent today. Until 1961, mental healthcare was not a covered health insurance benefit. Despite the Affordable Care Act (ACA) mandated parity, coverage is stringently limited and not affordable for many. Despite expanded coverage, mental health resources are insufficient to meet the U.S.'s needs and access to care is not equitably distributed. Marginalized groups—the poor, POC, and the LGBTQ+—who have the highest needs are, paradoxically, the least likely to receive care.

Research shows that within healthcare there is persistent implicit bias and discrimination toward people with mental disorders, who are likely seen as violent, incompetent, or just acting out, instead of people who are ill and vulnerable. The stigmatization of mental disorders, implicit bias, and discrimination are known contributors to people's reluctance to seek care. On the other hand, unlike hypertension and diabetes, the diagnosis and treatment of mental disorders tend to be complicated and fraught. Rarely, are there simple diagnostic tests and straightforward treatments, as with physical problems. Although psychotropic drugs work well in about 16% of the cases, that leaves 84% without adequate relief.

Recent studies are showing that people with a mental disorder are more likely to recover and lead productive lives when therapy includes the three Ps: supportive People in their lives, a safe Place to live, and a Purpose to get up every day.[30] Despite the effectiveness of the three Ps, these resources are not commonly available. They take money and providers to oversee coordination of care; they are outside healthcare's sanctioned treatment—drugs and surgery—and they are not covered by insurance. Instead, emergency departments are the default setting for patients in crisis. While the acute incident is usually resolved, the care is not optimal. Most emergency department staff don't have the skills and training to provide mental health care; the physical layout of an emergency department often adds to the patient's distress; and most need out-patient follow-up care, which the community may not have or the patient can't afford. Finally, because of the dearth of state and local in-patient facilities, patient who need in-patient care can wait days and even months in the local emergency department before a bed becomes available.

Mental disorders are strongly associated in the two structural determinants of health: SOCIOECONOMIC AND POLITICAL CONTEXT and SOCIOECONOMIC POSITION. Mental disorders are associated with inadequate economic well-being, inequities in accessing the community's resources, and social exclusion. These are significant stressors, which, when chronic, harm the mind, as well as the body.

Each year the American Psychological Association conducts a survey to study stress in the U.S.—its causes, and how people are responding both physically and mentally. Data from 2019 through 2023 surveys show that COVID-19 made long-standing problems worse, as noted by increases in the incidence of chronic diseases and mental health problems. In 2024, twelve trends the APA documented included "the ongoing crisis in mental health access, the trauma for women and LGBTQ+ individuals whose bodily autonomy is threatened by ongoing legislation, and the backlash against racial equity."[31]

While President Biden in his 2022 State of the Union message called to dramatically expand the supply, diversity, and cultural competency of mental health and substance abuse resources, it's not clear when that will happen. Due to inadequate treatment facilities, psychiatrists and other mental health providers, the ongoing mental health crisis continues to strain U.S. emergency rooms two years after President Biden's State of the Union message.

## Systemic Redesign

COVID-19 exposed and exacerbated the fractures in the system, that is, inequitable access to care and inequitable distribution of resources, as well as the mental models that drive health inequities (Figure 7.1). According to systems thinking, the more fragile the system, the more it amplifies the chaos in the environment. COVID-19 exposed and exacerbated healthcare's inequities. Because they were built into the system a long time ago, it's not fair to blame the original designers. However, it is fair to heed Einstein's warning, "You can't solve today's problems with yesterday's thinking." Today, most of healthcare's inequities, as well as its ineffectiveness and inefficiencies, are the result of "yesterday's thinking."

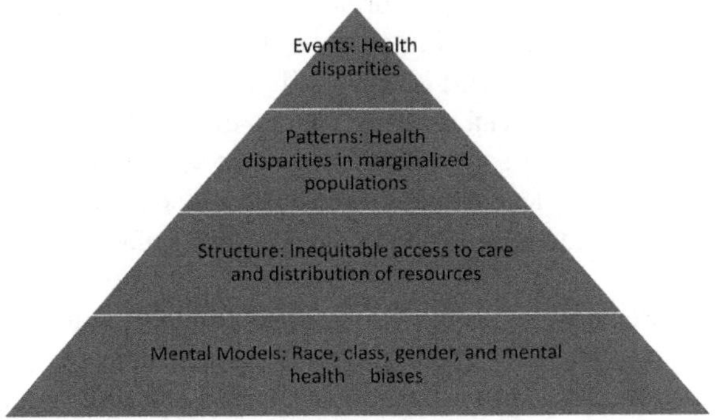


*Figure 7.1* Iceberg Model: Drivers of Health Inequities

In 2017, the Robert Woods Johnson Foundation offered four key steps to achieve health equity, which apply to mental and physical health:

1 **Identify important health disparities**. Many disparities in health are rooted in inequities in the opportunities and resources needed to be as healthy as possible. The determinants of health include living and working conditions, education, income, neighborhood characteristic, social inclusion, and medical care. An increase in opportunities to be healthier will benefit everyone but more focus should be placed on groups that have been excluded or marginalized in the past.
2 **Change and implement policies, laws, systems, environments, and practices to reduce inequities in the opportunities and resources needed to be as healthy as possible.** Eliminate the unfair individual and institutional social conditions that give rise to the inequities.
3 **Evaluate and monitor efforts using short- and long-term measures** as it may take decades or generations to reduce some health disparities. In order not to underestimate the size of the gap between advantaged and disadvantaged, disadvantaged groups should not be compared to the general population but to advantaged groups.
4 **Reassess strategies in light of process and outcomes and plan next steps.** Actively engage those most affected by disparities in the identification, design, implementation, and evaluation of promising solutions.[32]

At the 2023, Population Health Colloquium, Paul Keckley, an expert in healthcare policy and reform, compared the U.S. healthcare system to peer countries' systems and reportedly proposed the following changes to make the U.S. healthcare system more efficient, effective, and fair:

- **The other countries had global budgets for healthcare.** Those countries decided that "there's a fixed amount of money we're going to spend," Keckley said. "You think that's going to happen [here]"?
- **The other countries had national standards of care.** "There was a standard of care that the government oversaw," he said. "We don't [have that] … We let everybody determine what's appropriate care, and then we defend it."
- **The other countries made primary care the central form of care.** However, there was a caveat to that, said Keckley: "It wasn't [about] health *or* social services. It was health *and* social services, funded directly by taxes at 2.5 times what we spend in the U.S. on social services, and in which behavioral and physical medicine, prophylactic dentistry, and over-the-counter and prescription drugs were integrated into those models of primary health. That sounded pretty good to me."[33]

The solutions are known. It is not a secret that equitable solutions require policy changes. For a very long time, peer countries have healthcare systems that have much better outcomes but cost half as much. There's research suggesting "the U.S. spends less than other high-income countries on social services, such as child care, education, paid sick leave, and unemployment insurance, which could improve population health."[34] In contrast, one study showed the U.S. spending on social services is greater or similar to other OECD countries.[35] The most likely reason for the difference is wealthier peers are more equitably spreading the money spent on social services; whereas, in the U.S. spending on healthcare and social policies is uneven, reflecting the structural and historical policies of the region. Ironically, America's chief complaint—healthcare's soaring costs—is an obstacle to change. Healthcare is awash in money. Yet, our for-profit system and $4.5 trillion dollars are potent incentives for powerful special interest groups to protect their economic interests, that is, to optimize their part.

The other obstacle is trust. Healthy relationships are built on trust. According to systems thinking, relationships matter. Relationships are the "connecting" rods that hold a system's parts together by controlling the flow of information and resources from part to part. In systems thinking, healthy relationships assure the flow of information and resources are equitable and that no part benefits to the detriment of the whole. Healthy relationships reinforce *mutually* optimizing activities among the parts. However, where there's a lack of trust in human systems, the reaction of each part is to defend, protect, and strengthen itself. COVID-19 eroded trust, especially in the government and people's trust science. COVID-19 also left Americans anxious and politically polarized, further fracturing the U.S. healthcare system. Rebuilding trust is possible—but that requires time, discipline, and the commitment of all the parts to the health of the whole system.

## Questions for the Reader

The questions provide an opportunity to examine your own mental models and values and to imagine other stakeholders' beliefs, fears, and values.

1 Should all Americans receive equitable care? Why do you believe this; what might others believe?
2 Does being treated unfairly causes stress? Can too much stress affect health? Why; what might others believe?
3 If you need care, do you live in an area where healthcare resources are readily available? Should basic healthcare sources be available to all Americans regardless of where they live, who they are, and whether they can personally pay for care? Why; what might others believe?
4 In your experience have you, or someone you know, not received the needed care because of gender, race, or ethnicity, or economic status? If yes, what kind of care was not received? What was the health impact? How did it make you feel?
5 In your experience, are politicians, corporate lobbyists, and insurance executives interested in creating a more equitable healthcare system? Why; what might others believe?
6 Have you, or anyone you know, experienced unfair treatment by a healthcare provider? If yes, how did that make you feel? Did your heath suffer because of this treatment? If yes, what do you attribute the unfair treatment to … being a member of a minority group, gender, economic status? Something else?
7 If you are a member of a minority group, would you prefer being treated by someone who looks like you and has your cultural values? If yes, why? If no, why not?

8 Is it fair to doctors and hospitals that different insurances pay different amounts for the same kind of care and that patients have different out-of-pocket costs for that care, depending on the insurance? Why; what might others believe?
9 Do you know anyone who has not been able to access mental health services on a timely basis? If yes, what was the result of not getting care when needed?
10 What was the reason care was unavailable? Affordability, lack of providers, something else?
11 Does the U.S. need more mental health facilities and practitioners? Where should the money come from?
12 If all Americans should receive equitable care, whose job is it to redesign the U.S. healthcare system to produce more equitable care: the government; the health insurance industry; private, integrated health systems like CVS Health Corporation; other?

## Notes

1 Tada, J.E. Brainy Quote. https://www.brainyquote.com/quotes/joni_ereakson_tada_526391.
2 Health Equity in Health People. (2030). https://health.gov/healthypeople/priority-areas/health-equity-healthy-people-2030.
3 Grogan, C.M. (2023). *Grow and Hide: The History of America's Health Care State*. New York: Oxford University Press.
4 Craig, D.M. (2014). *Health Care as a Social Good: Religious Values and American Democracy*. Washington, DC: Georgetown University Press.
5 Institute of Medicine (US) Committee on the Consequences of Uninsurance. (2002). *Care without Coverage: Too Little, Too Late*. Washington, DC: National Academies Press.
6 Hoit, G., Wijeysundera, W., Hamad, D. et al. (2024, July 24). Insurance type and withdrawal of life-sustaining therapy in critically injured trauma patients. *JAMA Network*. https://jamanetwork.com/journals/jamanetworkopen/fullarticle/2821463.
7 American Hospital Association. (2023, May 17). Improving Health Care Access in Rural Communities: Obstacles and Opportunities. *Statement of the AHA for the Committee on Finance, Subcommittee of Health Care of the U.S. Senate. Obstacles and Challenges Facing Rural Communities*. https://aha.org/system/files/media/file/2023.
8 Americans in Rural Areas Don't Live as Long as Their Urban Counterparts. (2021, August 12). *UTMB News*. www.utmb.edu/news/article/utmb-news/2021/08/12/americans-in-rural-areas.
9 Saving Rural Hospitals, Overview. *Center for Quality and Payment Reform*. https://chqpr.org/Overview.html.
10 What Happens When a Hospital Closes? (2022, August 18). *Freakonomics MD*. https://freakonomics.com/podcast/what-happens-when-a-hospital-closes.
11 Schaefer, S.L., Mullens, C.L., & Ibrahim, A. (2023, April 4). The emergence of rural emergency hospitals: Safely implementing new models of care. *JAMA Network*. https://jamanetwork.com/journals/jama/issue/329/13.
12 Ducharme, J., & Wolfson, E. (2019, June 17). Your Zip Code Might Determine How Long You Live—and the Difference Could Decades. *Time*. https://time.com/5608268/zip-code-health.
13 Ducharme, J., & Wolfson, E. (2019, June 17). Your Zip Code Might Determine How Long You Live—and the Difference Could Decades. *Time*. https://time.com/5608268/zip-code-health.
14 https://www.cdc/gov/minorityhealth/racism-disparities/index.html.
15 Percent of People without Health Insurance in the United States from 2010 to 2022, by Ethnicity. (2023, August 31). *Statista*. https://www.statista.com/statistics/200970/.

16 Smedley, B.D., Stith, A.Y., & Nelson, A.R. (Eds). (2001). *Unequal Treatment: Confronting Racial and Ethnic Disparities in Health Care.* Institute of Medicine. Washington, DC: National Academies of Science Press.
17 The Economic Burden of Racial, Ethnic, and Educational Health Disparities in the U.S. (2018). *National Institute on Minority Health & Health Disparities.* www.nimhd.nih.gov/about/publications/economic-burden-health-disparities-US-.
18 Snyder, J.E., Upton, R.D., Hassett, T.C., Lee, H., Nouri, Z., & Dill, M. (2023, April 14). Black representation in the primary care physician workforce and its association with population life expectancy and mortality rates in the US. *JAMA Network.* https://jamanetwork.com/journals/jamanetwork.
19 Howard, J. (2023, February 21). Only 5.7% of US doctors are Black, and experts warn the shortage. *CNN.* https://cnn.com/2023/02/21/health/black-doctors-shortage-us.
20 2019 National Healthcare Quality and Disparities Report [Internet]. (2020, December). Rockville (MD): Agency for Healthcare Research and Quality (US). Figure 15, Registered nurses by race/ethnicity (left) and U.S. population racial/ethnic distribution (right), 2018. Available from: https://www.ncbi.nlm.nih.gov/books/NBK579359/figure/ch2.fig16/.
21 Hospital administrator demographics and statistics in the US. (2023, July 21). https://zippia.com/hospital-administrator-jobs/demographics.
22 Hiding in Plain Sight: The Health Care Gender Toll. *Deloitte-US.* https://www2.deloitte.com/content/dam/Deloitte/us/.
23 Walton, J. Black. (2020, October 16). Women's biggest health issue is the system. *Hopkins Bloomberg Public Health.* https://magazine.jhsph.edu/2020/black-womens-biggest-health-issue-system.
24 Walton, J. Black. (2020, October 16). Women's biggest health issue is the system. *Hopkins Bloomberg Public Health.* https://magazine.jhsph.edu/2020/black-womens-biggest-health-issue-system.
25 Gillespie, C. (2022, November 23). Major health disparities affecting the LGBTQ+ community. https://www.health.com/mind-body/lgbtq-health-disparities.
26 Mental Health by the Numbers. *National Alliance for Mental Illness.* https://nami.org/mhstats.
27 Fiorillo, A., & Sartorius, N. (2021, December 13). Mortality gap and physical comorbidity of people with severe mental health disorders: the public health scandal. *Annals of General Psychiatry.* https://annals-general-psychiatry.biomedcentral.com/articles/.
28 *WHO Highlights Urgent Need to Transform Mental Health and Mental Health Care.* (2022, June 17). https://www.who.int/news/item/17-06-2022-who.
29 Panchal, N., Saunders, H., Rudowitz, R., & Cox, C. (March 20, 2023). The implications of COVID-19 for mental health and substance abuse. *KFF.* https://www.kff.org/mental-health/issue/issue-brief.
30 Insel, Thomas. (2022). *Healing: Our Path from Mental Illness to Mental Health.* New York: Penguin Press.
31 American Psychological Association. (2024, January/February). 12 Emerging Trends for 2024. https://www.apa.org/monitor/2024/01/trends-report.
32 Braveman, P., Arkin, E., Orleans, T., Proctor, T., & Plough, *A.* (2017, May 1). What is Health Equity. *Robert Woods Johnson Foundation.* www.rwjf.org/en/insights/our-research/2017/05/what-is-health-equity-html.
33 Frieden, J. (2023, September 19). Want better health outcomes, check out what other countries do. *Medpage Today.* https://www.medpagetoday.com/meetingcoverage/phc/106393.
34 The Commonwealth Fund. (2021, August 4). New international study: U.S. health system ranks last among 11 countries; many Americans struggle to afford care as income inequality widens. https://www.commonwealthfund.org/press-release/.
35 Papapanicolas, I., Woskie, L.R., Orlando, D., Orav, E.J., & Jha, A.K. (2019, August 14). The Relationship between Health Spending and Social Spending in High Income Countries: How Does the US Compare? *Health Affairs.* https://www.healthaffairs.org/doi/101377.hlthaff.2018.05187.

# 8 Social Capital and Social Cohesion

## Relationships Are the Glue That Hold Systems Together

Relationships matter. Systems are networks of relationships in which people and materials interact to form a meaningful whole. All systems have definable boundaries, are composed of identifiable parts that are connected by networks of interlocking relationships, receive inputs from other systems in the form of resources and information, and generate outputs to the world outside its boundaries. Parts, inputs, outputs, boundaries, and relationships are key to understanding systems.

Systems can be as small as a family or as large as a solar system. In systems language, relationships connect the parts. Carrying information and resources, relationships are the glue that hold its parts together internally and connect them to other systems externally. In everyday language, healthcare's internal relationships are the roles of its various stakeholders and its policies, rules, and regulations. Together, they determine the types and distribution of resources among the stakeholders.

Although there are many types of relationships—romantic, work, situational, to name a few—there are two that deserve special mention regarding healthcare. Transactional relationships are businesslike, based on mutual benefit; transactional relationships are a kind *of quid pro quo.* Transformational relationships are the second important type. Just as transformation denotes positive change or evolution, transformational relationships are about vulnerability and mutual caring, support, and inspiration for becoming the best version of themselves the participants can be. Human relationships are not inert, like some kind of computer code, or gears in a machine. Human relationships are dynamic, waxing, and waning according to the ways people communicate and behave with each other.

## The Therapeutic Relationship

At the heart of all healthcare interactions is the therapeutic relationship between the physician and the patient. The best therapeutic relationships are those that are reciprocal—built on compassion, collaboration, trust, and respect. This therapeutic relationship has become more complicated over time. Historically, because of the asymmetrical power of scientific knowledge, physicians assumed a kind of

DOI: 10.4324/9781003538226-9

paternalistic responsibility for their patients. Then, the patient's role was passive—to seek competent care and follow the doctor's orders.

Since then, both parties' responsibilities have changed and become more complex. The physician's fiduciary responsibility is no longer solely to the patient. Today, the physician has obligations to his employer and the patient's the insurer, as well as the patient. Adding to the complexity, physicians are often expected to consider the cost of the treatment as well as its therapeutic value, especially if the patient is uninsured or under-insured. Having been designated a consumer, the patient also has new and more responsibilities, including participating in medical decisions regarding his own care, having good lifestyle habits, knowing his covered benefits and which providers are in his network, and shopping for the best quality of care at his affordable price.

Despite, the recent complexities, the best therapeutic relationships are those that are reciprocal—built on compassion, collaboration, trust, and respect. While patients assume their providers are technically competent, they want a physician who sees them, feels them, gets them, and who's got them. Generally speaking, for the patient, strong therapeutic relationships foster better health outcomes. Decades of evidence show wounds heal faster, diabetic complications are fewer, symptoms of depression are less, and adherence to prescribed therapies are better, to name a few of the benefits.[1]

When the relationship is reciprocal, it's rich in information. The physician is drawn into the quantifiable psychosocial world of the patient and the patient is drawn into the uncertain world of clinical decisions. Paradoxically, when limits are acknowledged both parties gain. Both the patient and physician know with greater clarity what is at stake. Trust is deepened and informed consent is more informed. Mutual feelings of competency and respect for the other pervade the relationship. The patient has more faith in the efficacy of the clinical decision and the physician's sense of accomplishment is greater. For physicians, there's increased psychological safety, less burnout, and more joy and meaning in their work. There's also more patient loyalty, more repeat business, and fewer malpractice lawsuits.

Like all interpersonal relationships, the doctor-patient relationship is a fluid process, continually influenced by a multitude of factors, especially the U.S. healthcare system itself, the culture of the workplace, and each party's prevailing emotional state. For physicians, hectic schedules, chaos, risk of workplace violence, and burdensome administrative and financial targets are well-known hindrances to the therapeutic relationship. Because these same hindrances are also well-known causes of physician burnout and are problematic in a time of physician shortages, the IHI has recommended "improving the joy in work" as the antidote to burnout.

## Joy in Work and the Quadruple Aim

Known as the *IHI Framework for Improving Joy in Work*, briefly, the Framework states "joy in work is an essential resource for healing"; joy in work is an emergent property arising from clinical and operational process improvement; improving joy involves everyone, with each level of the organization committed to improving what is theirs to fix.[2]

Improving joy in work is not about pizza parties nor yoga classes. It's about re-designing workflows that cause workplace stress, because stress is an impediment to therapeutic relationships. Advocating process improvement, the Framework points to the effects poorly designed clinical and operational processes have on the staff. Among the effects are a waste of time and resources, lower morale, staff anxiety and conflict, and patient dissatisfaction. Similar to W. Edward Deming's fourteen points, the Framework acknowledges nine elements that are inherent to improving clinical and operational processes. They are (1) physical and psychological safety, or an equitable and just environment free from harm; (2) meaning and purpose, or a sense of connection to one's profession and the organization's mission; (3) choice and autonomy, or flexible hours; (4) recognition and reward, or acknowledgement of one's contributions; (5) participative management, or shared decision-making; (6) camaraderie and teamwork, or social cohesion, trust and respectful relationships; (7) daily improvement, or continuous, proactive learning from mistakes, defects, and successes; (8) wellness and resilience, or work-life balance and self-care for mind, body, and spirit; and (9) real-time measurement, or regular monitoring and radical candor in assessments.[3]

Now known as the Quadruple Aim, joy in work is an addition to the popular Triple Aim—enhancing the patient's experience, improving population health, and reducing healthcare costs. The Quadruple Aim underscores the importance of caring for the staff by removing impediments to joy. Although the Aim is local—improving hospital clinical and operational processes—its concepts offer a method for improving the whole U.S. healthcare system, especially that systemic improvement takes all of us. Each level of society is involved.

### Social Isolation Is Deadly

The cardiologist Dean Ornish, M.D., has done more to call attention to intimate and social relationships as health producing than any other American physician. According to Dr. Ornish, "The need for authentic connection and community is primal, as fundamental to our health and well-being as the need for air, water, and food."[4] When authentic connection and community are absent, people do not flourish. For instance, babies kept warm, dry, and fed but isolated from the caress of human touch and voice were more likely to die than those who were talked to and played with by the staff of an orphanage.[5] Social isolation and loneliness increases the risk from dying prematurely from heart disease.[6] A nine-year follow-up study of Alameda County, California residents showed that after adjusting for socioeconomic status and poor health habits, those who were least socially connected were twice as likely to die from all causes as were those with family or social ties.[7]

People who are socially isolated and lonely are at increased risk—at levels comparable to smoking a pack of cigarettes a day—for premature deaths from all causes, including suicide. Anxiety, depression, dementia, and poor life style habits are strongly associated with social isolation and loneliness. The biological effects of loneliness and social isolation are measured by elevated pathological markers of stress—such as high blood sugar, high blood pressure, inflammation, high cholesterol—all of which are contributors to premature death.

According to a 2023 report by the U.S. Surgeon General, Dr. Vivek Murthy, the U.S. is in the midst of an underappreciated public health crisis: an epidemic of loneliness and social isolation, affecting people of all ages. Acknowledging that social bonds are a source of healing and well-being, as well as important to community resilience and prosperity, the Surgeon General's Advisory called for the U.S. to establish a National Strategy to Advance Social Connections. Among its recommendation is to "**Cultivate a Culture of Connection:** [Because] [t]he informal practices of everyday life (the norms and culture of how we engage one another) significantly influence the relationships we have in our lives."[8]

### Social Relationships Foster Health

Social bonds, or social connections, are not to be confused with being popular or having lots of social media "friends." Instead, social bonds refer to the coin of inclusion. Inclusion means a sense of belonging and being held in esteem; shared purpose and values; support for the bad times and celebration of the good; mutual aid; and safety in knowing you have access to the group's resources and are protected; and comfort in knowing you are cared for.

It's well known that social bonds are protective to physical and mental health. Simply speaking, there are reciprocal relationships among and between social bonds, positive emotions, the four "feel good" hormones—oxytocin, dopamine, serotonin, and endorphins—and health and well-being. The "feel good" hormones are powerful downregulators to the body's stress responses, making them immensely protective against many chronic diseases. They also upregulate the body's rest-relax-repair response. Producing happy, positive feelings, the four feel-good hormones reduce feelings of anxiety and stress, thereby, improving mental health. Of the four hormones, oxytocin is also associated with trust and love, feelings that foster social connections.

According to Barbara Fredrickson,[9] a leading researcher in the broaden and build theory of positive emotions, positive emotions do more than upregulate the body's relaxation response. Positive emotions foster healthy social relationships; oxytocin is associated with bonding, trust, and empathy. The four feel good hormones also increase creativity and resilience by broadening people's minds, opening them to new possibilities, new information, new relationships, and new social resources, which are key to healthy relationships and healthy systems.

### Social Capital and Social Cohesion

Social capital and social cohesion are related. Social capital is an umbrella term that refers to networks of social relationships that provide value to its members, individually and collectively. Social capital is built from trust, reciprocity, and mutual aid, which, collectively, enable network members to work together for their mutual benefit. A network is a group of inter-dependent people who have something in common. Networks vary in size and in purpose. Networks can be as small as a handful of friends, a family, or a work group; or as large as a corporation, a political party, or a country; or anything in between. Social cohesion, which comes from social capital, refers to the strength, or cohesiveness, of large networks. A function of trustworthiness, cooperation, and a sense of solidarity, social cohesion is the sense that we're all in this together so let's make it work for everyone.

Both social capital and social cohesion effect health, in multiple ways, which is the purpose of this chapter. Both are important personal and community resources. Both are fragile, can easily be destroyed, and take years to rebuild. Despite their fragility, it's widely known that social bonds are fundamental to health and well-being, and it is widely believed that strengthening social bonds and social cohesion within communities is important to improving health outcomes and reducing health inequities.

As the WHO[10] schematic shows (Figure 8.1) Social cohesion & Social capital arise at the intersection of Socioeconomic position and the Intermediary Determinants. This means that social capital and social cohesion are the products of material circumstances, such as gender, education, income and race, and psychosocial factors, such as emotional intelligence, likeability, and trust. The arrows go in both directions. For the individual, social capital signifies the coin of inclusion—friendships, a sense of belonging, mutual aid, and safety. For large networks, such as neighborhoods, ethnic groups, and communities, social cohesion signifies social stability—safety, access to the community's resources, collaboration and cooperation among and between asymmetrical groups.

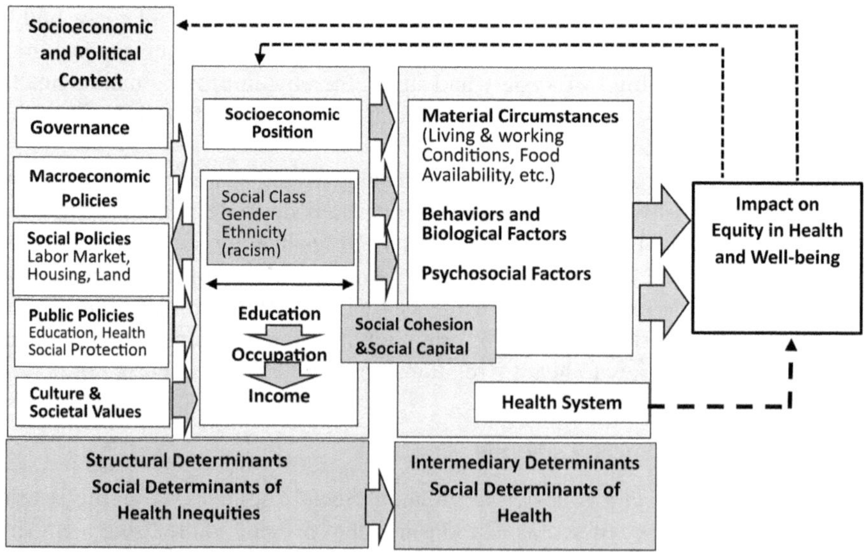


*Figure 8.1* WHO Social Determinants of Health

## Three Forms of Social Capital

Often referred to as the "glue" that holds societies together, social capital comes in three forms: bonding, bridging, and linking. *Bonding* refers to the value derived from positive connections between people—trust, reciprocity, and mutual aid—which allow people who are similar in social position to work together to achieve a common purpose and for their mutual good. *Bridging* refers to trust, respectful relationships, and mutuality between groups that are not similar in social position to work together for a common good. And, *linking* refers to trust, respectful relationships, and shared norms and cultural values between asymmetrical networks, that is, networks of differences in institutional authority, economic power, and so forth. Linking allows networks of people with a lower social position access to opportunities and resources controlled by the higher status group. Bonding and bridging are integral to social cohesion. Linking and bridging are integral to equity.

## The Health Producing Power of Social Cohesion

Social cohesion is protective to physical and mental health. The protective power of bridging social capital was documented in a famous cardiology study conducted in the mid-20th century in Roseto, Pennsylvania, a close-knit Italian-American community. During the seven-year period, the study discovered that no one under the age of forty-seven died from heart disease; men over sixty-five died from heart disease at half the rate of the U.S. population; and the death rate from all causes was 35% lower than rest of the U.S. Despite the community having all the normal lifestyle habits of the U.S. population—smoking, a high-fat diet, regular alcohol consumption, and working in toxic slate mines—the population was unusually healthy. The reason: The community was close-knit. The miners and the managers went to the same churches, bowled on the same leagues, lived in the same kinds of houses, and their kids went to the same schools. Sometimes known as the Roseto effect, high levels of bridging capital, or social solidarity, are health producing. Unfortunately, social solidarity of Roseto gradually eroded. By the early 1970s, family ties began loosening. Younger generations moved away and conspicuous consumption became the norm, causing the Roseto effect to fade. A follow-up study, twenty years later, showed that health status of this community mirrored that of the rest of the U.S. The protective effect of bridging had disappeared.

One of the earliest perspectives of the effects of social cohesion and health was provided by Emil Durkheim in his studies on suicide in the late 1890s. Known as the father of sociology, Durkheim believed that social bonds belong to the community and signify the health of the community. Studying the effects of rapid social change during the early stages of capitalism, Durkheim posited that the community itself is a complex entity. Like the metaphor of the chicken and the egg, Durkheim observed that the community acts on and through each person to influence the health status of each just as the health status of each person affects the overall health of the community. In his famous study on suicide, published in 1897, Durkheim concluded that the more integrated a person is into the social fabric, the less likely he is to commit suicide. In short, the more cohesive the social fabric, the fewer the suicides. Suicide, therefore, is not the result of a personal deficit, nor is it a psychological phenomenon. Instead, according to Durkheim, suicide is a social phenomenon. Like the proverbial dead canary in the coal mine, suicide is a symptom of the breakdown of the cohesiveness of society and social instability.

Using Durkheim's perspective, it's not an accident that the opioid epidemic arose in Appalachia, a region once replete with well-paying mining and manufacturing jobs, blue collar jobs that required a strong back but not a college education. As jobs disappeared, social cohesion frayed, then fractured. However, the physical pain of old injuries remained, compounded by the emotional pain from loss of jobs and social status. To numb the pain, opioid prescriptions were sought and written. Due to the combination of aggressive marketing, Purdue Pharma greed, and false claims that Oxycontin was not addictive, people became addicted. Families fell apart. As social cohesiveness fragmented, the region experienced higher numbers of opioid deaths than other regions of the U.S., especially among less educated, White males under fifty.

Although death rates vary by state and region, the continuing rise in deaths of despair—suicide, drug, and alcohol abuse—indicate a frayed social fabric, one that is too frayed to be protective. This suggests that the best efforts to mitigate deaths of despair are not downstream treatment centers—although important—but are upstream, at improving employment opportunities, especially for men living in these regions.

As the above examples show, bridging capital fosters social cohesion, which benefits everyone's health. Conversely, when bridging capital is lacking, social cohesion disintegrates, and the overall health of the community deteriorates. Finally, bridging capital is a significant contributor to resilience and disaster recovery from large natural disasters, whether Hurricane Katrina or the disastrous wildfire in Hawaii. Bridging capital often comes from the heart. While waiting for the official responders to natural disasters, numerous studies show community members jump in to do whatever is needed. Bridging capital ties together people of different social status, fosters inclusiveness, and enables people of asymmetrical status to share resources and information. In political jargon, bridging capital is the willingness to "work across the aisle." That Congress increasingly refuses to work across the aisle doesn't bode well for social cohesion.

Much like adding money to a savings account, bridging capital can be deliberately increased. Basically, this means expanding one's social circle to include people not like you to work together toward a common goal. Expansion includes joining associations, clubs, civic and professional groups, or becoming involved in volunteer activities. Bridging capital accrues when groups that are not similar in social position work together for a common good, such as a food coop in Riverton, Wyoming or Philadelphia's Beat the Heat initiative, which provides heat relief resources for neighborhoods.

### Linking Social Capital Offers Low Status Groups a More Equitable Access to Resources

Linking social capital refers to networks of trusting, respectful relationships between people of different social status with the purpose of the lower status group gaining either access to or a more equitable distribution of resources. Of the three forms of social capital, linking has special value in that it provides access and connection to power structures and their resources. Like bridging, linking social capital fosters a more equitable distribution of a community's and a country's resources and opportunities.

Flint, Michigan was once a thriving industrial city. Now, it's a low-income, predominantly African American community, best known for its public health water crisis. Caused by social injustice, bad economics, and bad decision-making, the quasi-resolution of the water crisis exemplifies the power of effective linking. Briefly, because the story has been told many times, the water crisis began in 2014 when the city manager of Flint changed the city's water supply from one source to a cheaper source. Inadequate water treatment and testing exposed about 100,000 people to Legionnaires disease and toxic levels of lead. Lead exposure in children is known to damage the brain and nervous system, delay growth and development, and cause learning and behavioral problems that can affect a child for the rest of his life.

The resolution, which took years and two dozen lawsuits, came from disparate groups linking together—the Hurley Children's Clinic, Dr. Mona Hanna-Attisha, a local pediatrician, local citizens and clergy, the Michigan American Civil Liberties Union (ACLU), and national water scientists, to name a few—to use the leverage of the courts and the state get safe tap water for the citizens of Flint. Although almost all the issues have been resolved, water safety—like everywhere—remains an ongoing concern.

Another example of linking is Medicaid expansion by putting it on the ballot. To overcome state legislature opposition, grassroot groups in six states—Oklahoma, Idaho, Maine, Nebraska, Missouri, and Utah—worked hard to put Medicaid expansion on the ballot, giving tens of thousands of low-income people in their states access to healthcare. Similarly, in reaction to the Supreme Court's decision to overturn Roe vs Wade, voters in several states have elected to add abortion protections to their constitutions or rejected proposals to further limit abortion access.

## Social Capital, Social Cohesion, and COVID-19

Sociologists debate whether social capital is a property that belongs to the individual or to the network. One side posits that social capital belongs to and is a phenomenon of the network. According to this perspective, social capital is the amount of participatory potential, which refers to shared values, trust, and mutual cooperation, that resides within and is used for the benefit of everyone within the network. The other side posits that social capital is generated by and belongs to the individual, but is not equally available to everyone. According to the belongs-to-the-individual side of the argument, social capital is derived from where one fits in the social determinants of health (SDOH) structural category Socioeconomic Position and is for the individual to use, typically, for his own advantage. Each side of the debate has its merits and describes an aspect of human behavior that the other side does not.

The acute phase of the COVID-19 pandemic lasted roughly between January, 2020 and May, 2022. Beyond the pandemic's immediate and personal threats of death, long haul symptoms, and economic loss, COVID-19 also infected the social fabric. Trust decayed, social bonds degraded, social cohesion splintered, mutual cooperation vanished, and the U.S. became more polarized than any time since the Civil War. The immediate effects of this lack of social cohesion were concerning. Over one million Americans died, proportionately more than in other wealthy countries. COVID-19 exacerbated health inequities for the poor and People of Color and engendered a growing mental health crisis. Adding insult to injury, COVID-19 also helped trigger the politicization of healthcare and the loss of trust in science.

As handling of COVID-19 became politically polarized, frontline staff went from heroes to villains. As the polarization increased, bridging capital degraded. Trust, respectful relationships, and mutuality between patient and provider faltered. Too many families and patients seemingly took comfort in inflicting their fears and frustration on the frontline staff. The painful irony is that the frontline workers, who were putting their own lives at risk, became the subjects of increasing violence and harassment. (This misfortune happened to other "essential workers," as well.) By mid-2021, COVID-19 was associated with unprecedented numbers of physicians and nurses committing suicide. By mid-2021, more than half of America's physicians, nurses, and other frontline staff reported feeling burned out and ready to leave healthcare.

One way or another, all Americans were affected, especially prior to the development of the vaccine when social isolation, lockdowns, and travel restrictions were used to control the spread of the virus. As the pandemic spread, supply chains broke; the economy contracted; people hoarded. Many non-essential employees were laid off or furloughed while upper income workers worked from home. Schools were closed, replaced with virtual learning from home, adding to familial stress. As a result, depression, anxiety, domestic violence, child abuse, and drug and alcohol abuse all increased, symptoms of pandemic-related stress.

During times of crisis and widespread stress, with its concomitant widespread anxiety, effective communication tends to be challenging. In the U.S., the governmental response to COVID-19 was fraught with challenges, starting with a novel virus about which very little was known at the onset of the pandemic. Other challenges ranged from uncooperatively and poorly coordinated responses from various federal agencies, conflicting agendas between the business and scientific communities, to the easy use of social media to spread outright misinformation and lies. Adding to the confusion and fear were the overt, public disputes between President Trump and Dr. Anthony Fauci, his chief medical advisor for COVID-19. The net result was a loss of social cohesion as exemplified by a confused and mistrusting public, whose frayed social bonds were further eroded by the political polarization that continued to escalate as the pandemic wore on.

Bereft of a national policy, the country splintered, with each of the fifty states developing its own COVID-19 response plan. Global supply chain issues and the lack of national coordination led to a spike in hospital costs as states and large hospital systems competed against each other for personal protective equipment, ventilators, staff, and other resources. Bidding against each other, the states and large systems perpetuated a vicious cycle that inexorably drove up healthcare costs.

Pretending the virus stopped at state borders and voted, or that the pandemic was a hoax, the plans varied widely from state to state. Many of the plans were driven, not by science, but by the fear, anger, and grief associated with COVID-19's impact on the state's economy, as well as the personal hardships the public experienced. Ideological differences and distrust of the federal government added to fragmentation's toxic stew.

Social cohesion is built from a willingness to work together for mutual benefit, and willingness to work together is built from trust. Just as most cars run on gasoline, social systems, like healthcare, run on information. The effectiveness, efficiency, and fairness of any healthcare system depend upon whether people trust the information entering and flowing through the system; whether there's transparency; whether the information is distributed to the right parts at the right time; and whether the information stays free of corruption as it flows from part to part.

The net results of COVID-19's effect on trust and loss of social cohesion was the death of a million Americans—with red states having almost three times more deaths than blue states.[11,12] COVID-19 was more than a wakeup call. It was a mirror reflecting a healthcare—a social system—unable to mount an effective and efficient response to COVID-19. It was a mirror reflecting long-standing systemic unfairness that is harmful to the health of the poor and People of Color. It was a mirror reflecting that mental health cannot be separated from physical health and that personal health cannot be separated from the social stability, national security, and economic stability of the U.S. It was a mirror clearly showing that health is more than a consumer product. Reflecting the lack of social cohesion, COVID-19 reflected a fragmented, fractious republic whose citizens were unable, or unwilling, to trust and to cooperate to protect the health and well-being of everyone.

## Social Capital Is Key to Healthy People, Healthy Communities, and Healthy Systems

Human beings are created to live in community. The Roseto effect is one way of saying cohesive communities are healthy communities. Social capital is a major contributor to the cohesiveness of a community. It is a measure of the quality of the relationships within the community, that is, it's a measure of trust and cooperation, which are vital to the well-being of the whole.

Because relationships are the "glue" that holds together social systems, social capital is important for the maintenance of healthy social systems. When people deeply care about the well-being of that system, their behavior supports the caring, and trust goes along for the ride. However, when the bonds of relationships are weak or frayed, trust flies out the window. The parts struggle to optimize themselves, and the system is unstable. Unstable systems amplify environmental chaos; whereas, stable systems are resilient and dampen environmental chaos.

## Social Capital Can Be Increased

Social capital is well named. Like having discretionary money, social capital provides a sense of personal physical and psychological security. For social systems, like healthcare, social capital represents the quality of relationships among the parts that determine the efficiency, effectiveness, and equity of the system. The good news is social capital can be deliberately increased, like adding money to a savings account. Building social capital is a choice—something people can chose to do or not. Because it is a function of relationships, social capital is increased by strengthening relationships. The bad news is it's not easy for it involves the rewiring of our brains.

Neuroscientists have shown human brains are plastic. Because they are plastic, they can be deliberately rewired. Briefly, the wiring of our brains reflects our lived experiences, our interactions with others, and our habitual thoughts and feelings about ourselves, our jobs, our society, and the people and things we like and don't like, to name a few. Our brains are wired to scan for safety and connection and for danger. Although, we habitually give more attention to danger than to safety and connection. This is, in part, because scanning for danger is teleologically lifesaving, a remnant from being "tiger food" eons ago. The other part is habit. Due to a myriad of experiences, starting in childhood, most of us have wired our brains to be more sensitive to danger than to safety. And, social media algorithms are designed to keep us perpetually on edge, if we let it.

As a result, for most of us, our brains and nervous systems are wired so that our minds and bodies are in a habitual state of low-level stress, a state of contraction, and defensiveness. Stress hormones narrow our perception and compromise our ability to trust and scan for safety and connection. Because stress hormones prepare us to fight or flee, the status quo may feel safer than the risk of bridging or linking with a stranger.

Building social capital involves rewiring our brains and nervous system to become more comfortable with risk. Building social capital is similar to a toddler learning to walk. Each time he loses his balance, falls, gets up, and takes a few more steps, he's rewiring his brain and nervous system. With enough practice, the circuits become so strong that walking is effortless. Building social capital takes similar practice. We are training our bodies to be calm and relaxed and our minds to scan for safety and connection in novel situations. Training ourselves to be calm and relaxed does not mean being a doormat or passive, agreeing with everyone, or waiving our own rights and needs. Instead, calm and relaxed has overtones of being confident and creative.

When we're relaxed, the four build and broaden hormones are upregulated. As a result, we are less reactive. We're open to new information, new experiences, and new opportunities, which are critical to finding common ground and building social capital. It's a tall order that takes deliberate and ongoing practice. Fortunately, there are all kinds of ways to retrain the brain to be more in a habitual state of low-level relaxation, ranging from mindfulness and breath practices, to apps, to finding joy in work between social support, and physical activity, among others.

The benefits to being in a habitual state of low-level relaxation are many. First and foremost is better personal physical and mental health. Second when we are calm, others perceive us as safe. A sense of safety can reduce the emotional temperature of a hot situation and can evoke the "build and broaden" state in others. Third, arising from this state are mutual curiosity, creativity, and caring, needed for building all three forms of social capital. Finally, information is more freely shared among the group. The multiple perspectives enable people to see problems as others see them, which mitigates the propensity to optimize one's part and often leads to more holistic solutions.

That said, the bonds of social capital are fragile and not all relationships can be strengthened. Greed, fear, anger, ego, and the benefits of the status quo are impediments to building social capital. All parties in the relationship have to *want* to change their minds and to work *together* for the good of the whole. Because life is full of surprise and change, social bonds generally need ongoing renewal and strengthening, otherwise they won't last. Social capital can take a long time to accrue but can be quickly destroyed by exploitation, betrayal, loss of trust, and carelessness.

**Calls for Cohesiveness**

Recommendations to overcome the multiple weaknesses that COVID-19 exposed and exacerbated in the U.S.'s public health system were addressed in a 2022 report from the Bipartisan Policy Center. "Advocating for a strong and effective national public health system that can improve health outcomes, advance equity, and respond to a myriad of possible emergencies,"[13] the Bipartisan Policy Center report called for a more centralized national public health system that is coordinated at the federal level. The recommended priorities included strengthening the nation's public health infrastructure; updating the antiquated data systems; and creating a top-down, federal structure that can coordinate actions among federal, state, local, and tribal health departments, healthcare providers, and medical suppliers. Adequate funding was also a priority. It's too early to tell the outcome of these recommendations.

Focusing on the growing influence of state governments on health and the widening gap in health disparities across the 50 states, Steven H. Woolf, M.D., concluded that "[t]he COVID-19 pandemic removed any doubt that state policies can affect health outcomes."[14] He did not mean this in a positive way. Starting in the 1990s, America's shorter life expectancy and higher burden of disease began worsening and noticeably varying by state. For instance, Mississippi has the lowest average lifespan of 74.6 years, whereas, Hawaii has the highest at 80.7 years. According to Woolf, the widening gap in health disparities across the 50 states cannot be explained by racial differences but are due to the effects of political priorities and policy choices that widened the gap in "education, wages, taxes, social programs, corporate profits, wealth inequality, and infrastructure."[15] Based on the disproportionate COVID-19 death rates in states that resisted public health recommendations and the widening gap in health disparities across the 50 states, Woolf suggested that "The nation should also reflect on federalism and decide whether it wants health policy to come in 50 varieties, considering the Constitution and

Tenth Amendment granted public authority (i.e. 'police powers') to the states … Although state governments have the right to set their own path and policies, the public should decide whether life expectancy should be part of the experiment."[16]

## Drivers of Fragmentation

COVID-19 is an acute, communicable disease caused by the SARS-CoV-2 virus. Acute refers to diseases that have an abrupt onset, are short lasting, and often need urgent care. Communicable means that the disease can be transmitted by a virus or bacterium to other people, which scientists refer to as community transmission. Communicable and community have much in common. Both come from an old French word meaning to share, join, unite—literally, to make common. Community, however, has a more specific meaning—joint ownership.

In theory, communicable diseases should unite people. Community transmission should inspire people to work together to reduce the risk of spreading the disease and animate them to share resources for their own and others' protection. Instead, COVID-19 polarized Americans, exacerbating the fractures in an already fractured system (Figure 8.2). By early 2022, COVID-19 had spread so widely that nearly 60% of U.S. adults and 75% of children had COVID-19 antibodies in their blood. Although 60% of U.S. adults had COVID-19 in common, it did not strengthen the bonds of community. Instead, like a house divided against itself, pandemic-stressed Americans worked against each other rather than uniting against a common enemy. At every level of society, the bonds of community were degraded by some combination of social isolation, distrust, disaffection, and denial. To make matters more fractious, the glue which holds society together—civility, respect, and cooperation—were egregiously replaced by harassments and death threats. All levels of society experienced these threats—from Dr. Fauci, public health officials, doctors caring

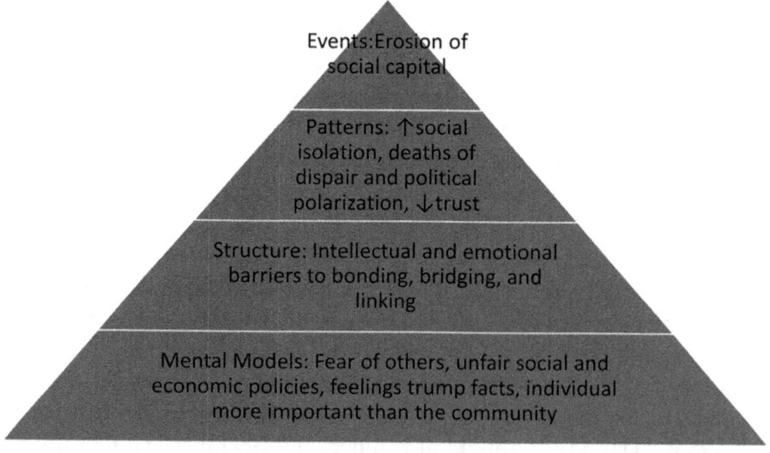


*Figure 8.2* Drivers of Fragmentation

for COVID-19 patients, to school board members. Even airline flights were disrupted by disagreements over wearing masks.

The questions are: "Why was the U.S. healthcare system unable to mount an effective response to COVID-19"? "Why did Americans work against each other and not together to defeat a common enemy"? and "Why did the public mistrust science and expert knowledge"? The answers can be found in the mental models from which the U.S. healthcare system has evolved.

Dig deep enough, and one finds the mental models that configure the U.S. healthcare system are based on values and beliefs that are rooted in the Age of Enlightenment. It was a time of radical progress that drove the ascendency of the natural science and economics. The assumptions arising from this period are (1) nature can be controlled, (2) subject and object are independent entities, (3) objective data is more valid than subjective thoughts and feelings, (4) the mind is separate from the body, (5) humans are rational, self-interested, and independent of each other, (6) technology is value-free and morally neutral, and (7) problems are best solved using linear, reductionistic thinking and complex decisions are best left to experts.

For a very long time, these assumptions drove progress, prosperity, and longevity. A good thing, indeed. Today, however, the limitations of these theories and concepts are showing as problems arise that cannot be resolved within Enlightenment constraints. Social conditions have changed, as have the burden of disease. Life is more complex and the effects of the social, political, and geophysical environment are real and greater than was imaginable 300 years ago. Technology is not morally neutral; it hasn't made everyone better off. Enlightenment's assumptions help drive civic fragmentation and distrust, as well as the feelings that profits are more important than people. Today, the limitations of Enlightenment's concepts are apparent in a healthcare system that is inefficient, ineffective, and inequitable.

Because of the configuration of the U.S. healthcare system, Americans entered the pandemic with poorer health status and more health disparities than their wealthier counterparts. While universal access to healthcare is important, the better health status of peer countries is largely attributed to the protective benefits of their stronger and better social safety nets. In contrast, access to healthcare in the U.S. is fragmented by type of insurance, geography, and social position. It's unknown how many adults didn't seek care for COVID-19 because they couldn't afford it. Unfortunately, when care was finally sought it was usually more intensive and more expensive care. Furthermore, millions of Americans don't have sick leave for America is one of very few wealthy countries that doesn't have universal sick leave. Bereft of paid sick leave and unable to afford staying home, millions of American with COVID-19 went to work and infected their coworkers—even though isolation is key to preventing its spread. Staying together as a community—strong social safety nets, universal health care, and universal sick leave—were important to other wealthy nations' effective response to the pandemic. In contrast, the U.S. didn't do so well. Operating on principals from the Age of Enlightenment, the U.S. championed the individual with his inalienable rights and self-interest over the welfare of the community.

The main reason the response of the U.S. was less effective than other countries—including poorer countries—was trust! A 2022 study published in Lancet showed that countries that higher levels of trust in the government and other citizens had significantly lower rates of infection. Although age, followed by GDP per capita, and obesity contributed to lower death rates, trust was the most important factor of all [infection and death].[17] This study is in agreement with decades of other studies that indicate that when people trust their government and other citizens, they are more likely to comply with public health measures, such as masking and social distancing, and expect others to do the same. The study also suggested that other countries' higher vaccine rates were directly associated with the public's trust in the government and other citizens.[18]

Trust is a shared resource. It is generated by the community. Trust enables the community to do what individuals cannot. Years ago, Ichiro Kawachi and Bruce Kennedy showed that *social capital*—trust, reciprocity, and mutual aid—are strongly correlated with health and mortality. To over simplify a bit, when people were asked, "Can most people be trusted—or would most people try to take advantage of you if they got a chance"? both disaffection and distrust highly correlated with income inequality and overall mortality.[19]

There's no doubt the Centers for Disease Control and Prevention (CDC), with its frequently changing and sometimes confusing and contradictory messages, and the lack of a unified federal response contributed to the public's mistrust of science and the government. However, the novel virus, itself, contributed to the messaging problems. With a new virus, scientists had very little information to guide decisions to stop its spread, forecast its effects, and develop effective treatments. It takes time to learn how the virus spreads, determine effective containment, best treatment methods, and develop vaccines for prevention.

On the other hand, two causes of distrust are rooted in two mental models. The first is the mental model that champions the rights of the individual over the welfare of the community. The second is the mental model that places more value on objective data than subjective feelings, even though how someone *feels* about a fact generally determines how he will act. If people don't feel safe, they automatically act defensively. Comments such as, "I don't want that mRNA in my DNA"; "there's a chip in the vaccine that will track my movements"; and my people were part of the Tuskegee experiment" indicate that vaccine hesitancy, for instance, arises from not feeling safe. Perhaps, trust would have eroded less had the messengers taken into account the public's emotional state, better emphasized that knowledge about COVID-19 was evolving, and provided a sense of hope and unity—that we're all in this together—during this difficult time. The reason President Franklin Roosevelt's famous speech, "We have nothing to fear but fear itself," continues to resonate is because the message was hopeful, honest, and called Americans to work together to defeat a common enemy.

Simply speaking, our social and personal encounters with the external world trigger an internal stream of biological events that our computerlike minds instantaneously reduce to one decision: Am I safe or in danger? In a split second, the body translates a cascade of neural, endocrine, and immune reactions into emotions. Despite Enlightenment's claim that we are rational beings, in truth, we are not. Nobel prize winning behavioral economists and psychologists have shown that our decisions are seldom rational but emotional. Thus, who's going to believe scientific data when one's emotions are screaming, "I don't feel safe"? Driven by emotions, we then use data, or the echo chamber of our favorite news organization or computer site, to justify our decisions to protect ourselves.

Ineluctably, COVID-19 showed that healthcare is more than a consumer product: It's a social good. The mental model that configures healthcare—that posits that the self is an independent entity, separate from its community, and is imbued with inalienable rights—has fostered selfishness. Purportedly independent from each other and the things we make, the mental models condition us to externalized blame. With our penchant for objectivity, it is easy to blame healthcare's failings on forces outside ourselves, such as Wall Street, special interest groups, or corporate lobbyists—or even healthcare itself.

Having externalized the things we make, it's easy to sidestep our own culpability as evidenced by accepting as normal: (1) a healthcare system that is fragmented by insurance type and population group, (2) the high incidence of health disparities among the poor and People of Color, and (3) the rights of the individual trump the welfare of the whole. COVID-19 clearly demonstrated that when individual "freedoms" aren't balanced by the community's needs, social capital evaporates and the whole community suffers. During the first two years of COVID-19, over a million Americans died and the national economy contracted because Americans were unable, or unwilling, to work together.

To summarize, the U.S. has the most expensive healthcare system in the world, with costs rising annually. It's the only system in the developed world that doesn't cover everyone. It's the only system in the developed world that is for-profit. Despite its high costs, the U.S. healthcare system's access, health outcomes, and equity are second tier compared to peer countries. Although COVID-19 further exacerbated the U.S. healthcare system's long-standing inefficiencies, ineffectiveness, and inequities, the silver lining in the pandemic's storm is it highlighted the need for an American healthcare system that works for everyone.

## Questions for the Reader

The questions provide an opportunity to examine your own mental models and values and to imagine other stakeholders' beliefs, fears, and values.

1. How much of your health is dependent upon your relationships—with your family, your friends, your community?
2. If something were to happen to you, would anyone know? In the case of an emergency, who would come to your aid?
3. In your experience are social isolation and loneliness on the rise in the U.S.? Are social isolation and loneliness harmful to health? Do you have a network of friends and a supportive family? Should your doctor be responsible for assessing your health risk of loneliness and intervene, if necessary? If someone is lonely and/or socially isolated who should be responsible to help the person cultivate social bonds? The person, his family, a social agency, healthcare, the government, other? How should these remedies be paid for? Why do you believe this; what might others believe?

4 Are diseases of despair—suicide, substance abuse, and their related deaths—due to a lack of social cohesion? Who should be responsible to prevent deaths of despair, the individual, healthcare, the government, the business community, some combination of these groups linked together? Why; what might others believe?
5 How much of your health is dependent on your community? Do the actions of others in your community and/or the actions of your state and national governments affect your health? Why; what might others believe?
6 What kinds of resources are available in your community for you? Do you have access to healthy foods, good education, healthcare, recreation, and a safe and clean environment? Are the same resources available to the poor and People of Color? Who do you believe should be responsible for adequate resources in your community? The local government, state, and/or federal government, community social service agencies, the churches, the hospitals, each family or person should be responsible for themselves? Why; what might others believe?
7 Have you ever used your social position to bridge or link with others to improve the health of someone else? Describe your experience.
8 How much of your health is having a voice in community decisions that affect your health? If your neighbors, or others, have more or less voice, does this affect your health? Why; what might others believe?
9 COVID-19 damaged the public's trust in healthcare and in science, although the public's trust in healthcare has been steadily decreasing since the mid-1960s.[20] Thinking about the future, if the U.S. were to experience another pandemic, who would you trust? The federal government, your state government, your physician, other? Why would you place your trust there?
10 Thinking about the future, who would you trust to reform healthcare? The federal government, your state, the health insurance industry, the hospital industry, the AMA, the pharmaceutical industry, large corporations like Amazon and CVS, other? Why; what might others believe?

## Notes

1 Trzeciak, S., & Mazzarelli, T. (2019). *Compassionomics: The Revolutionary Scientific Evidence That Caring Makes a Difference.* Pensacola, FL: The Studer Group.
2 Perlo, J., Balik, B., Swensen, S., Kabcenell, A., Landsman, J., & Feeley D. (2017). IHI Framework for Improving Joy in Work. *IHI White Paper*. Cambridge, MA: Institute for Healthcare Improvement. (Available at ihi.org).
3 Perlo, J., Balik, B., Swensen, S., Kabcenell, A., Landsman, J., & Feeley D. (2017). IHI Framework for Improving Joy in Work. *IHI White Paper*. Cambridge, MA: Institute for Healthcare Improvement. (Available at ihi.org).
4 Ornish, D., & Ornish, A. (2019). *Undo It!: How Simple Lifestyle Changes Can Reverse Most Chronic Diseases.* New York: Ballantine Books. p.196.
5 Harmon, K. (2010, May 6). How Important Is Physical Contact with Your Infant? *Scientific American.* https://www.scientificamerican.com/article/infant-touch.
6 Rogers, K. (2023, December 24). Loneliness or Social Isolation Linked to Serious Health Outcomes, Study Finds. *CNN.* https://www.cnn.com/2023/06/19/health-loneliness.
7 Berkman, L.F. & Kawachi, I. (2000). Social networks, host resistance, and mortality: A nine-year follow-up study of Alameda County Residents. *American Journal of Epidemiology*. 241 186–204.

8 New Surgeon General Advisory Raises Alarm about the Devastating Impact of the Epidemic of Loneliness and Isolation in the United States. (2023, May 3). https://www.hhs.gov/about/news/2023/05/03/new-surgeon-general-advisory-raises-alarm-about-devastating-impact-epidemic-loneliness-isolation-united-states.html.
9 Fredrickson, B. *The Science of Happiness, Theory*. https://pursuit-of-happiness.org/history.
10 A Conceptual Framework for Action re the Social Determinants of Health, Discussion Paper 2. (2010, July 13). *WHO*. https://www.who.int/publications/i/item/9782941500852.
11 Chappell, B. (2023, July 25). Republican's excess death rate spiked after COVID-19 vaccines arrived, a study says. *NPR*. https://www.npr.org/2023/07/25/1098543849/.
12 Wallace, J., Goldsmith-Pinkham, P., & Schwartz, J.L. (2023, July 24). Excess death rates for Republican and Democratic registered voters in Florida and Ohio during the COVID-19 pandemic. *JAMA Network*. https://jamanetwork.com/journals/jamainternal.
13 Armooh, T., Barton, T., Burgon, A., Donnellan, J., & Harootunian, l. (2021, June 29). Positioning America's public health system for the next pandemic. *Bipartisan Policy Center*. https://bipartisanpolicy.org/report/preparing-for-the-next-pandemic/.
14 Woolf, S.H. (2022, March 11). The growing influence of state governments on population health in the United States. *JAMA Network*. https://jamanetwork.com/journals/jama/fullarticle/2790238.
15 Woolf, S.H. (2022, March 11). The growing influence of state governments on population health in the United States. *JAMA Network*. https://jamanetwork.com/journals/jama/fullarticle/2790238.
16 Woolf, S.H. (2022, March 11). The growing influence of state governments on population health in the United States. *JAMA Network*. https://jamanetwork.com/journals/jama/fullarticle/2790238.
17 Aleem, Z. (2022, February 3). Study shows trust in the government helps fight the pandemic. *MSNBC*. https://www.msnbc.com/opinion/study-shows-trust.
18 Aleem, Z. (2022, February 3). Study shows trust in the government helps fight the pandemic. *MSNBC*. https://www.msnbc.com/opinion/study-shows-trust.
19 Kawachi, I., & Kennedy, B.P. (1999) Health and social cohesion: Why care about income inequality. In I Kawachi, B.P. Kennedy, & R.G. Wilkinson (Eds.) *The Society and Population Health Reader: Income Inequality and Health* (Vol. 1). New York: Press, pp. 195–210.
20 Baker, D.W. (2020, December 15). Trust in health care in the time of COVID-19. *JAMA Network*. https://jamanetwork.com/journals/jama/fullar.

# 9 Choices

## Americans Have Lost Confidence and Trust in Their Healthcare System

Americans have lost confidence and trust in their healthcare system. The following three 2023 headlines say it all. Health insurance cost jump to nearly $24,000 for a family of four, a 7% increase from 2022.[1] *Diagnostic errors linked to nearly 8000,000 deaths or cases of permanent disability in US each year, study estimates.*[2] While "there's actually less than a 0.1% chance of serious harm related to misdiagnosis after a healthcare visit … [n]early 40% of the bad outcomes are linked to errors in diagnosing five conditions: stroke, sepsis, pneumonia, blood clots in veins, and lung cancer."[3]

The third headline, *Trust in healthcare is declining, and the costs to providers is rising*,[4] captures America's dilemma. The word dilemma originally referred to a rhetorical device in which an opponent was presented with two equally undesirable alternatives. Hence, the phrase "caught on the horns of a dilemma." Whichever horn was chosen, the argument was lost. One horn of the bull was as damaging as the other. A dilemma means either choice makes things worse.

Behind the trust headline was a survey asking adults "whether their healthcare system's highest priority was serving patients or generating profits." Two thirds said profits! A dilemma, indeed. One horn is the public's valid concerns regarding the affordability of healthcare; the other, however, is the hospitals' equally valid financial concerns. Most American hospitals had negative profits margins between 2020 and 2022, the time of COVID-19. Although hospital margins began recovering in 2023, 40% of U.S. hospitals were still losing money in 2024. According to Kaufman Hall, the significant damage is to the lowest performing 20% of rural hospitals where operating margins are much lower than struggling urban hospitals. This level of financial performance is not only unsustainable but makes the continuation of under-reimbursed services, like obstetrics, impossible.[5] The dilemma is clear. If there's no margin, there's no mission. To cut costs is to cut services. On the flip side, to raise prices is to raise the number who can't afford healthcare.

The irony is while Americans are paying more for healthcare and many hospitals are barely surviving, insurance companies are making out like bandits. In 2022, the top four insurance companies posted profits ranging from the high of $20.6 billion for UnitedHealth Group to the low of $6 billion for Elevance.[6] When

DOI: 10.4324/9781003538226-10

insurers celebrate record profits and when 30% of rural hospitals and over 200 other hospitals are at the risk of closure,[7] there's something obviously wrong with the U.S. healthcare system.

Study after study and headline after headline show a steady loss of confidence and trust in the U.S. healthcare system, which corresponds with rising costs, inadequate benefit coverage, narrowing networks, and concerns about quality and fairness. Because the public's concerns have risen to the attention of Congress, it's likely that healthcare reform will be on the national political agenda, following the 2024 election.

### What Do Americans Want?

What do Americans want from their healthcare system? They want care that is affordable, convenient, timely, easily accessible, and is safe and high quality. They want to have health insurance if they lose their job, don't have a job, work part-time, or are unable to work. They want to be able to count on their covered benefits being adequate for their health needs and staying the same from year to year. Americans don't want their doctor or hospital or pharmaceutical benefits change annually, depending on the plan their employer purchased that year. They want affordable care. They don't want to shop for the best price, or double-check to see if the ambulance, anesthesiologist, or ED doctor is in their network—especially if they are in the midst of a medical emergency. They want to choose their own doctors and hospitals and they want their doctor, not their insurance company, to decide the kind of care they need. They'd also like covered benefits for dental, vision, hearing, and mental disorders, and maybe long-term care. What Americans want has been known for a long, long time. However, healthcare reform has always been fraught and fragmented.

### Why Is Reform So Fraught?

In a *New York Times* editorial, Paul Krugman once wrote, "One of the truly amazing and depressing things about the health reform debate is the persistence of fear-mongering over 'socialized Medicine,'" to which a reader replied, "another amazing and depressing thing is the persistence of an ignorant and misinformed public."[8] The cry of "socialized medicine" has long been used by special interest groups to trick the public into fearing they'd have to pay more in taxes, not be able to choose their own doctor or hospital, have longer wait times, or that universal healthcare is a "Communist plot." Going as far back as President Truman's proposal for universal healthcare, the American Medical Association (AMA) used the fear of "socialized medicine" to defeat Truman's proposal, claiming—inaccurately—that doctors would lose their autonomy to the federal government. Truman never forgave the AMA for misrepresenting his proposal.

The blunt answer is that healthcare reform involves distributive justice. Ironically, the public's chief complaint—healthcare's soaring costs—is an obstacle to change. Healthcare is awash in money; $4.5 trillion dollars is a potent incentive for powerful special interest groups to protect their economic benefits at weaker stakeholders' expense. Every time healthcare reform rises to the top of the national political agenda, powerful special interest groups flood the public with an overwhelming amount of misinformation, deliberately designed to resonate with the public's fears. For example, distilled from multi-million-dollar ad campaigns against the Affordable Care Act (ACA) were memes of "death panels," "socialized medicine," "I'm not your ATM," and "government overreach." Repeated and amplified through the echo chamber of social media, these memes resonated with those who feared the ACA would cost them more but provide less coverage. The memes also resonated with those who feared others' gain would be their loss. Ironically, many of the fears were not misplaced. After each "reform" attempt the U.S. healthcare system, overall, did not become more efficient, effective, nor equitable, but succeeded in increasing American's costs.

## Three Models to Choose From

Dilemmas present two equally undesirable alternatives. The way out of a dilemma is to go above and beyond the two false, forced choices and find other, better options. One of the benefits of social capital is it creates space for new information and new opportunities to emerge. Better options tend to be available if they are looked for. The good news is there already are better healthcare systems—systems that provide more efficient, effective, and equitable care. The U.S. does not need to reinvent the wheel. Around the time U.S. legislators were debating the Affordable Care Act, a Washington Post correspondent named T.R. Reid[9] set out to learn why other wealthy countries have healthcare systems that were more efficient, effective, and equitable than ours. Reid found that there are four models of healthcare systems, three of which are more effective, efficient, and equitable than the U.S. healthcare system.

In his global quest, Reid visited five wealthy, industrialized countries—Canada, France, Germany, Japan, and the Great Britain—to learn what made their systems so much better. Speaking to doctors, government officials, policy analysists, and patients, Reid discovered that these countries have in common a non-profit healthcare system and a commitment to providing necessary health care to all of their citizens. In short, everyone is included and no one is left out.

These countries consider healthy citizens to be integral to a strong and economically productive country. Recognizing that sickness and trauma can't be planned for, like buying a vehicle, that sooner or later everyone will get sick, and that one person's sickness affects the community, as well as the family, peer countries put all their citizens in the same risk pool. Risk is not segregated as in the U.S. In these wealthy countries, everyone pays something, either through taxes, like Canada and Great Britain, or through a dual financing system of taxes and private health insurance, like Germany and Japan. Bottom line, other wealthy countries understand that, overall, it is less costly, healthier, and more equitable for everyone to have access to the same kind of care and to share the costs of this care among the entire population.

At the end of his quest, Reid concluded, despite local variations, every country has a health care system that fits one of these four models, period. None of the models are perfect, but three of the four produce better health outcomes at about half the cost of the U.S. healthcare system. Reid named the four models the BEVERIDGE, the BISMARCK, the NATIONAL HEALTH INSURANCE, and the OUT-OF-POCKET model.

## A Closer Look at Reid's Four Basic Models

The BEVERIDGE model is named after William Beveridge, the social reformer responsible for Britain's National Health Service. Commonly known as the National Health Service (NHS), the BEVERIDGE model has been used in the United Kingdom since 1948. Like the American Veterans Administration, the NHS is financed by taxes. Hospitals and clinics are owned and operated by the NHS. Most doctors are NHS employees, although there are private practitioners who bill the government. Patients are never billed since care is free at the point of care; however, most adults have to pay for prescription drugs, although the price is nominal, about $10 in 2022.

Costs are controlled through several levels of regulation. At the policy level, the government establishes price controls, expenditure caps, and the types and location of services. At the local level, access to care depends upon the number and types of physicians and facilities. The doctor determines the patients' medical needs at the clinical level. The bottom line is the entire population is guaranteed access to a predetermined level of care. Equity of care, access, and cost control are the principal values of this model.

The key characteristics of this model are public financing and public facilities and providers. Great Britain, Spain, and most of the Scandinavian countries use this model, as does the U.S. Department of Veteran Affairs. The model is not perfect. A significant downside is care is financed through taxes, hence the risk of underfunding. The NHS was once considered the best healthcare system in the world. Since 2010, its funds have been steadily cut, leaving the NHS in crisis with too few hospital beds, too few providers, and very long wait times. As a result, people who can afford to are buying private insurance and turning to private care, which simply accelerates a vicious circle and a race to the bottom. In 2022, the British cost for healthcare was $5,493 per person compared to the U.S. cost of $12,555, according to Organization for Economic Cooperation and Development (OECD) data.[10]

The BISMARCK model is named for the Prussian Chancellor Otto von Bismark, who created a welfare state to facilitate the unification of Germany in the 19th century. In this model, healthcare is part of Germany's general social insurance program, which includes healthcare, pensions, unemployment, work-related injuries, and long-term care. Providers and facilities are usually private. Care is paid for through a multi-payer, private insurance system, known as sick funds, which are financed jointly by employers and employees through payroll taxes.

In Germany, everyone has health insurance. No one loses his health insurance if he loses his job. Smaller employers and their employees don't pay more than larger employers and their employees. Insurance plans cover everyone with the same set of benefits. Although the insurance is private, insurers cannot make a profit. Rates are set and the funds are tightly regulated by a quasi-governmental board that includes members of the public. Physician and hospital costs are negotiated annually and are set according to a fixed set of covered services, limited by law to services that are economically viable, sufficient, necessary, and meaningful.

The BISMARK model is based on the belief that society is responsible for the well-being of its members. The entire population is guaranteed access to a predetermined level of care. Equity of care, access, and cost control are the principal values of this model. The key characteristics of this non-profit model are quasi-private insurance and private providers and facilities. In 2022, the German costs for healthcare were $8,011 per person.[11] Germany, France, Belgium, and Japan are some of the countries using this model.

The NATIONAL HEALTH INSURANCE model, also known as the "single payer" or Canadian model, has elements of the BEVERIDGE and BISMARCK models. The single payer model uses private providers and facilities who are paid by a single-payer, publicly funded insurance program. Hence, its popular name, "single-payer." With few exceptions, all citizens are covered for a fixed set of "essential" care, including preventive care, costing Canadians $6,319 per person in 2022.[12]

Canadians control costs by virtue of little overhead and administrative simplicity. The cost savings is significant, since it's estimated that if the U.S. were to cut its spending on billing overhead to match Canadian levels, the cost saving would be enough to provide first dollar coverage for all Americans.[13] The Canadian government's ability to negotiate lower pharmaceutical and durable medical good prices is also important to controlling costs. The key characteristics of this non-profit model are public insurance and private providers and facilities. Its principal values are equity of care, access, and cost control. Canada is the exemplar of the single payer system; however, Taiwan and South Korea also use this model, as does traditional Medicare.

Reid's fourth model is the OUT-OF-POCKET model, which is found in countries too poor or disorganized to have an established healthcare system. In poor countries, there are not enough doctors and hospitals and the available few are found in the nation's capital and other large cities. There is no health insurance, little or no government funding to pay for care, and those who can't pay are not treated—unless they are lucky enough to have access to doctors from international charity organizations. The key characteristics of this entrepreneurial model are private providers and facilities and no insurance. Most third-world countries use this model, as do, unfortunately, uninsured Americans.

### Benefits of the Three Universal Models

The three universal models are non-profit and none of them is perfect. Each of the three—British, German, and Canadian—is unique. Each uses a different combination of public and private responsibilities for the delivery and/or payment of care. However, all three models share several important commonalities that make them more efficient, effective, and equitable than the U.S. healthcare system.

First, they are all affordable. Second, all citizens are included and everyone—regardless of age, employment, ethnicity, income, pre-existing conditions, or where they live—has access to care. Third, every citizen has access to the same package of covered services. Fourth, payment doesn't vary; for each covered service, doctors and hospital are paid the same. Finally, employers are freed of a significant business expense, health insurance. With U.S. employers paying an average of $8,435 per worker in 2023, the savings to American businesses would be huge.

## Benefits to Patients

All citizens are included and everyone—regardless of age, employment, ethnicity, pre-existing conditions, or where they live—has access to care. And, every citizen has access to the same package of covered services. Regardless of whether the insurance premiums are paid for by taxes, by employer/employee contributions, patients have little, if any out-of-pocket costs. There are no "surprise" bills and the patient is not expected to shop for care at the best price. With little out-of-pocket costs, health outcomes are better because there's no reason for citizens with universal care to avoid or delay care because of costs concerns. Because drugs cost significantly less than they do in the U.S., drugs are taken as prescribed, compared to the 8% of Americans who don't fill a prescription, skip doses, or take less than prescribed because of costs. Drug prices are controlled by a variety of governmental policies and insurance covers the cost.

Universal care eliminates financial fears. No one loses access to care if they lose their job with its subsidized health insurance. No one goes bankrupt over medical bills. How many Americans can pay the 20% their insurance doesn't cover on a million-dollar medical bill, an amount that is not uncommon. About fifty percent of Americans have unpaid medical bills. Although most go unpaid, the pressure to pay causes many to lose their life savings, empty their children's education fund, go bankrupt, have their wages garnished, or a lien placed on their house. Furthermore, medical debt contributes to poor health outcomes. Shame and fear of more debt keep people from seeking care when needed, and the stress of medical debt harms the body's capacity to heal and contributes to adverse health outcomes. Universal coverage eliminates the toxic financial stress that interferes with healing and recovery.

## Benefits to Doctors

Universal coverage models are good for physicians, too. While some physicians complain that they'd like to have the income American physicians have, in all three models, physicians are paid well. That said, each model, as well as each country, has its own formula for negotiating payment to the physicians. With the exception of Great Britain, countries using these models have more physicians per population than does the U.S. Their physicians generally work shorter hours than American physicians and have more clinical autonomy. Physicians and hospitals aren't financially punished for caring for low-income patients. Physicians don't experience moral injury, which refers to the psychological harm that comes from a violation of one's core values. Moral injury stems from knowing what level of care the patient needs but unable to provide it because the patient doesn't have insurance or his insurance won't pay for it.

Medical school debt is not a burden in countries that have universal healthcare. The average medical school debt for American doctors is about $200,000; debt for Canadian doctors is around $100,000; and Europeans leave medical school with little or no debt because it is free or highly subsidized. Because these countries subsidize medical schooling, they have more physicians practicing medicine than in the U.S. Because care is universal, a worker seriously injured on the job, a person made quadriplegic by a car accident, or a family whose baby was born with cerebral palsy don't attempt to afford ongoing care by suing a doctor or hospital. As a result, with these three models, malpractice insurance costs and malpractice claims are minimal. As a result, the incentive to practice costly "defensive medicine" is also minimal.

## Benefit to Hospitals

Although all three models use global budgets, each peer country has its own formula for determining payments to hospitals. The result is hospitals know up front how much they will receive to pay for care as well as for capital construction. Because reimbursement is standardized, there's no cost shifting and no need for "safety net" hospitals. In peer countries, 40% of their hospitals aren't at risk of going broke because reimbursement is less than the costs.

Like herding cats, hospitals in the U.S. have to deal with over 1,000 insurance companies, each of which has multiple kinds of plans, each with unique requirements. Because there's no standardization among the insurance companies nor their plans, hospitals are forced to have armies of registration, coding, clinical documentation, and billing staff just to meet multiple insurers' billing and prior authorization demands. The lack of standardization is costly. Americans pay more than four times the amount Canadians to process the patients' bills. Similarly, American doctors submit about four times more medical documentation than physicians in other countries do.

Fragmentation and the lack of standardization affect hospital budgets. For example, reimbursement from Medicare and Medicaid is so low it usually doesn't cover the hospital's actual cost of care. On the other hand, not every private insurer pays the same but varies according to what the hospital can negotiate with the insurance company. Typically, insurance companies that cover a large percentage of the hospital's patients use their leverage to negotiate lower payments, which could be even lower than Medicare's. While this benefits the insurer, it doesn't benefit the hospital nor is the "cost savings" passed on to the patient.

## Global Budgets

In contrast to the U.S. system, the purpose of the three models is to keep people healthy, not make a profit for investors. All three models use a global budget to control costs. Global budgets are similar to a household budget. At the start of each year, a predetermined pool of monies is earmarked to pay for healthcare. This pool of monies is tied to some arbitrary criterion, such as a fixed percentage of GDP or a fixed annual growth rate.

Global budgets are a commitment to both economic efficiency and a predetermined level of healthcare for every citizen. Similar to a household budget but on a national scale, global budgets involve several layers of control. At the national level, the government or a statutory entity establishes price controls, expenditure caps, and the types and location of services.

At the local level, access to care depends upon the number and types of physicians and facilities, which are, generally, matched to the size of the population and its health needs. At the clinical level, for all three models, the *doctor* determines the patients' medical needs. In contrast, American doctors have lost much of their autonomy to insurance companies. In the U.S., medical care is determined more by reimbursement policies than the physician's clinical judgment. The insertion of the insurance company into the therapeutic relationship has made physicians responsible for balancing the patients' medical needs with the payers' financial requirements. This insertion has compromised the physicians' authority, their ability to be an advocate for the patient, and has undermined the doctor-patient relationship, the heart of health care.

Prices are controlled by the government or the governing board, which, after negotiations, sets the prices doctors and hospitals can charge. Price controls mean that every doctor and every hospital are essentially paid the same price for the same service. For example, in 2020, the average charge for hip replacement surgery in Canada was about $10,500,[14] compared to around $39,000 in the U.S. where there can be a ten-fold charge difference from hospital to hospital.[15] This eliminates cost shifting, since prices are controlled and all providers and hospitals are paid the same.

Total, annual costs are controlled through expenditure caps. Just as a household sets aside fixed amounts of money to be spent on food, recreation, and so forth, expenditure caps refer to the predetermined amount of money the country will annually spend in the aggregate for various types of service delivery, such as cardiology, preventive care, etc. To prevent the maldistribution of services—such as one small town having four MRIs and no obstetricians—global budgets also control the location and distribution of services.

The beauty of a global budget is that cuts in one area are justified on the grounds the money will be spent on other, higher-priority services; whereas, in the U.S., cuts in one part of the system become the profits of another. With global budgets, cost shifting to increase profits isn't an option. A global budget isn't perfect. There are complaints, regardless of how the money is allocated. For example, healthcare in the U.K. is underfunded; U.K. citizens complain that advanced technology is not readily available; and doctors complain of low wages. Canadians complain of long wait times and underfunded rural areas. Germans, on the other hand, complain that they sometimes have out-of-pocket costs and their doctors complain that they don't make as much money as American doctors. Despite the complaints, all three models guarantee the entire population access to a predetermined level of care that is better, fairer, and much less expensive than the American model.

## Today's Challenges, Regardless of the Model

Twenty years later, Ezekiel Emanuel, M.D., a respected medical ethicist and policy expert, wrote, *Which Country Has the World's Best Health Care?*[16] Ezekiel compared the U.S. healthcare system with ten other countries—Australia, Canada, China, France, Germany, Netherlands, Norway, Switzerland, Taiwan, and Great Britain. Some of the countries were chosen because Americans were familiar with their healthcare system and some were chosen to expand the discussion to include the unfamiliar, providing opportunities to learn. Because all ten countries have some form of universal healthcare at costs less than the U.S.'s, Emanual's goal was to learn what works best in each system and could apply here.

Briefly, Emanuel discovered there's no best system; all have trade-offs. All control costs, but in different ways. No system is perfect; some do better at somethings and worse at others. No system is a "plug and play"; each fits within its historical antecedents and cultural values. And, all, including the U.S., are facing a common set of challenges:

1 Cost pressure—citizens want more care but object to higher taxes and premiums to pay for it
2 High and rising cost of pharmaceutical drugs
3 Unnecessary and low-value care
4 Care coordination between hospitals and out-patient services for patients with chronic diseases
5 Mismatch between healthcare delivery and the population's chronic health care needs, in other words, a mismatch between delivery and the social determinants of health
6 Provision of mental health
7 Provision of long-term care and how to pay for it.[17]

## The American Healthcare System Is Fragmented

When it comes to healthcare, the U.S. is unlike other wealthy countries in three significant ways. First, all other wealthy countries have *one* model for everyone, which is simpler and less costly to administer. Second, everyone has access to *affordable* healthcare through some kind of insurance, whether the insurance is paid for by taxes, or by a combination of public/private funds. Finally, everyone has the same package of covered services and all physicians and hospitals are, generally speaking, paid the same for the same care.

In contrast to other wealthy countries that have one *uniform* system, the U.S. healthcare system is a conglomerate of all four models. For example, medical care for military veterans uses the British model. Traditional Medicare for senior follows the Canadian model, and employer-subsidized health insurance follows the German model. The out-of-pocket model applies to Americans without employer-subsidized health insurance and are too young to qualify for Medicare or not poor enough to qualify for Medicaid. Because it's a conglomeration of competing systems, U.S. healthcare costs can only be shifted, not controlled.

Unlike other wealthy countries, healthcare in America is a for-profit system. Other wealthy countries do not have investor-owned hospitals, clinics, or large physician practices that are subject to the corporate imperative of quarterly economic growth. In other wealthy countries, healthcare is a social good, not a commodity to be bought by those who can afford the sticker price. For these countries, healthy citizens are considered integral to a strong and productive country. These countries understand that it is more effective, efficient, and equitable to give all citizens access to the same kind of care and to share its costs among the entire population.

The American public has been taught to fear universal healthcare will raise their taxes. The reality is that Americans already pay a massive tax for healthcare. Paid by a combination of employer and worker, the average annual family premium of $23,968 is a massive tax—only the "tax" goes to private insurance. Considering that, in 2021, American spending on healthcare is $12,914 per person, whereas the comparable average of similar wealthy countries was $6,125,[18] a tax increase for universal healthcare does not compute. According to a Washington Post article, "health insurance costs raise the average effective tax rate on American labor from 29% to 37%."[19] Tax dollars are already the single largest funding source for healthcare in the U.S., but Americans are not getting their money's worth.

Longer wait times are another popular reason the public cites against universal healthcare. Here, too, the facts do not support the belief. Data from countries with universal care show that these three models produce wait times that are similar or better than the U.S. model. For example, according to the OECD data, the percentage of patients reporting they got a response from their regular doctor on the same day ranged from a high of 33% in Canada and 28% in the U.S. to a low of 13% in Germany and 12% in Switzerland. Wait times for appointments to specialists and for non-emergent surgeries, the U.S. also performed worse than other wealthy countries.[20]

Despite the public's fears that universal healthcare means the government, not the patient, would choose which doctors and hospitals patients could use, the fears are false. With all three universal coverage models, the patients choose their own doctors, hospitals, labs, pharmacies, etc. In the U.S., commercial health insurance companies and Medicare Advantage with their "narrow networks" and "preferred provider organizations" control which doctors, hospitals, labs, and pharmacies Americans can use. None of the three universal models permits such restrictions.

All three models provide all citizens with equal access to a standard benefit package. With all three models, healthcare is efficient, effective, and equitable. Everyone has access. Everyone can afford healthcare for themselves and their families. Because care is affordable, there are no medical bankruptcies. Because care is affordable no family has to rely on crowd-funding or community spaghetti dinners to pay out-of-pocket medical bills. Because care is affordable people don't choose die at home instead of calling an ambulance because they can't afford the medical bill. Because care is affordable and available, women with breast cancer don't wait for the cancer to become an open wound before they seek care, and if they don't have insurance, they don't have to "shop" for a hospital that provides charity care. Because care is affordable people don't have to choose between medicine and food.

## Medicare for All

Believing that healthcare is a universal right Senator Bernie Sanders made Medicare for All part of his 2016 presidential campaign. Since then, he has renewed his push for universal healthcare through his proposed Medicare for All Act of 2023. Briefly, the Act proposes a single-payer, national health insurance that covers everyone in America and is free at the point of care. The proposed insurance is tax-based, eliminating networks, premiums, deductibles, and surprise bills. Pharmaceutic drug costs would be capped at $200 per year. The proposed legislation offers more expansive coverage than traditional Medicare and Medicare Advantage, including dental, vision, hearing, mental health and substance treatment, as well as home and community-based long-term care.[21]

The proposed legislation restructures the U.S. healthcare system, making it more equitable, efficient, and effective. By including everyone, the system is more equitable. By expanding coverage to include mental as well as physical health, for there is a strong inter-dependent relationship between physical and mental health, the system is more effective. By making healthcare free at the point of delivery, the system is more efficient—at least for patients.

The challenge, of course, is for reimbursement to cover the cost of care, which neither traditional Medicare nor Medicare Advantage currently do. Ironically, the other challenge is the public's chief complaint—healthcare's rising costs. Healthcare is awash in money—$4.5 trillion is a potent incentive for powerful interest groups to protect their economic benefits at the expense of weaker groups. While $4.5 trillion is certainly enough to share, it doesn't make the political task any easier in a culture that values wealth and champions the self.

## Just "Do It"—the U.S. Doesn't Have to Reinvent the Wheel

We know what can be done. We don't need to reinvent the wheel to reform the American health care system; there are three already proven models from which to choose. Whichever model is chosen, it won't be perfect and there will be trade-offs. However, comparison data show that peer countries' universal healthcare systems are more effective, efficient, and fair than ours.

For the U.S. to have a healthcare system that is more efficient, effective, and equitable than the current system, Americans should not only pick one of the models that has already been proven to work but, *equally important*, improve it. The data and examples are available. According to a Commonwealth blog,

> [It's] time for a new conversation. We must move beyond the arguments that have dominated the discourse for decades and instead look to the successful approaches of other countries. We can achieve universal coverage, invest in public delivery systems, and broaden our understanding of health care to include preventive services, public health initiatives, and the social drivers of health. These will make more of a difference than a simple change to a single-payer system.[22]

Universal healthcare is not a panacea. It does not automatically correlate with better health outcomes. Universal healthcare means that all citizens have access to healthcare and care that is free, or nearly free, at the point of delivery. While lessening the economic fears associated with trauma or a chronic disease is significant, universal healthcare is not likely to significantly improve overall health outcomes. This is because health outcomes and burden of disease are more closely associated with where a person lives and his socioeconomic status than access to healthcare. Even with universal healthcare, a person's zip code will still matter to some degree.

## Questions for the Reader

The questions provide an opportunity to examine your own mental models and values and to imagine other stakeholders' beliefs, fears, and values.

1 Using your own experience, following a health incident, did the outcome meet your expectations, was access to care easy and convenient, was it affordable?
2 Have you ever had to wait more than three days to see your primary care doctor or wait several months to see a specialist? If yes, how long did you have to wait? Would you pay more to cut to the front of the line? If yes, how much more?
3 Peer countries have proven that universal care, with one reimbursement method, and a global budget to control costs generate a healthcare system that is more efficient, effective, and equitable than the U.S.'s. Which of the three universal models would you pick and why? Knowing that none of the models is a "plug and play," what implementation problems do you foresee with your chosen model? How would you improve the model to best fit the needs of the U.S. population? Why; what might others think?
4 The 2023 Medicare for All legislation by Senator Bernie Sanders proposes a universal healthcare system that offers *comprehensive* coverage, including dental, vision, hearing, and community and long-term care support, eliminates co-pays and deductibles with the exception of some prescription drugs, prohibits commercial insurers to sell policies that duplicate benefits, and allows individual state to offer additional benefits.[23] Why would you support or not support this bill; what might others think?
5 If you prefer the current for-profit U.S. model instead of one of the universal models, why do you prefer to keep the current model? What might others think?
6 If the U.S. adopted some form of universal healthcare, which of the following would you want as a covered benefit and why? (1) preventive care, (2) curative, (3) rehabilitative, (4) palliative, (5) behavioral, (6) vision, (7) dental, (8) pharmaceutical drugs, (9) long-term care. How would these benefits be paid for?
7 In some peer countries patients can purchase private supplemental insurance to cover extra amenities and benefits, avoid wait times, and see physicians not covered by the national program. If the U.S. adopted some form of universal healthcare, do you think that those who can afford it should be able to purchase private supplemental insurance for extra benefits and amenities? Why; what might others believe?

## Notes

1 Rising health care costs have driven health insurance premiums to $24,000. (2023, October 18). Kffhealthnews.org. https://kffhealthnews.org/morning-breakout/rising.
2 McPhillips, D. (2023, July 19). Diagnostic errors linked to nearly 800,000 deaths or cases of permanent disability in US each year, study estimates. *CNN*. https://edition.cnn.com/2023/07/19/health/.
3 McPhillips, D. (2023, July 19). Diagnostic errors linked to nearly 800,000 deaths or cases of permanent disability in US each year, study estimates. *CNN*. https://edition.cnn.com/2023/07/19/health/.
4 Jarrard, D. (2023, October 7). Trust & consequences. *Jarrard Inc*. https://jarardinc.com/...2023/10/trust-consequencs.
5 The numbers behind the national hospital flash report. (2024, February 21). *Kaufman Hall*. https://www.kaufmanhall.com/insights/thoughts-ken.
6 Thomas, N., & Emerson, J. (2023, March 7). Large health systems vs payer profits in 2022. *Becker's Payer Issues*. https://www.beckershpayer.com/payer/large-health.
7 Dyrda, L. (2023, May 22). 646 hospitals at risk of closure, ranked by state. https://www.beckershospitalreview.com/finance/646.
8 Krugman. P. (2009, July 28). Why Americans hate single-payer insurance. *New York Times Web Archive*. https://archivenytimes.com/krugman.blogs.nytimes.
9 Reid, T.R. (2009). *The Healing of America: A Global Quest for Better, Cheaper, and Fairer Healthcare*. New York: Penguin Press.
10 Reid, T.R. (2009). *The Healing of America: A Global Quest for Better, Cheaper, and Fairer Healthcare*. New York: Penguin Press.
11 Reid, T.R. (2009). *The Healing of America: A Global Quest for Better, Cheaper, and Fairer Healthcare*. New York: Penguin Press.
12 Reid, T.R. (2009). *The Healing of America: A Global Quest for Better, Cheaper, and Fairer Healthcare*. New York: Penguin Press.
13 Abrams, A. (2020, January 6). The U.S. spends $2,500 per person on health care administrative costs. Canada spends $550. Here's why. *Time*. https://time.com.5779772.
14 CJRR Annual Report: Hip and knee replacements in Canada 2021–2022. (2023, September 28). *Canada Institute for Health Information*. https://www.cihi.ca/en/cjrr-annual-report-hip-and-knee-replacements-in-canada.
15 Lewis, S. (2020, September 8). How much does hip replacement cost? www.healthgrades.com/right-care/hip-replacement/how-much-does-hip-replacement-cost.
16 Emanuel, E. (2020). *Which Country Has the World's Best Health Care?* New York: Hatchette Book Group.
17 Emanuel, E. (2020). *Which Country Has the Best Health Care*. New York: Hatchette Book Group. pp. 10–14.
18 McGough, M., Telesford, I., Rakshit, S., Wager, E., & Amin, K. (2023, February 9). How does health spending in the US compare to other countries? *Peterson-KFF Health System Tracker*. https://www.healthsystemtracker.org/chart.
19 Ingraham, C. (2019, October 16). Americans already pay a "gigantic" hidden health care tax, economists say. *The Washington Post*. https://www.washingtonpost.com/business/2019/10/16.
20 Waldrop, T. (2019, October 18). The truth on wait times in universal coverage systems. https://americanprogress.org/truth.
21 Medicare for All 2023: Executive Summary. (2023). *Office of U.S. Senate Bernie Sanders*. https://berniesanders/com/issues/medicare-for-all.
22 Carroll, A. (2024, May 16). Rethinking health care from a global perspective: American complexity. *Commonwealth Fund*. https://www.commonwealthfund.org/blog/2024/.
23 Text-S.1655-118 Congress (2023–2024): Medicare for All Act. https://www.congress.gov/bill/118-congress/senate-bill/1655/text.

# 10 Healing

## A Call to Heal

In the early 20th century, when the U.S. healthcare system was in its infancy, the American naturalist, John Muir, writing about his first summer in the Sierra's, observed: "Whenever we try to pick out anything by itself, we find it hitched to everything in the universe." The quote is a reminder that life is complex, astonishing, and composed of an orderly arrangement of mutually interdependent parts. His words are also reminders that the whole can never be reduced to a collection of independent parts. The whole is unique—it is always more than the sum of its parts.

Drilling down from the universal to the particular, Muir's poetic words describe the organic nature of human systems, such as the U.S. healthcare system. It, too, is an orderly arrangement of interdependent parts that affect each other for good or ill. Each part has a definite role to play, but to fulfill its unique role each part depends upon the other parts to function properly. When all the parts of healthcare function properly, it is a productive and healthy system.

Like the human body, the healthcare system can become ill and fail. To use the human analogy, with serious physical illnesses, the body's vital organs can begin to fail. Since vital organs support each other, the failure of one causes the other organs to work harder, until they, too, begin to fail. Like the cascading effect of organ failure, the unaffordability of healthcare continues to seriously damage major parts of the U.S. healthcare system. For instance, according to a 2023 survey, more than half of adults with health insurance have trouble affording healthcare, causing many to avoid or delay care because of costs, even though delays or lack of care made people sicker. Struggling with costs, a growing part of the public avoids healthcare; however, hospitals are also struggling to stay in business. Hospitals compensate by expecting staff to do more with less, leading to staff burnout. Since insurance doesn't always cover the cost of care, hospitals also compensate by raising their rates. This triggers private insurance to raise the cost of their premiums, which triggers businesses to pass more of the cost of insurance to their employees, which causes more people to avoid healthcare. As with physical organ failure, the failure, if not reversed, can be fatal.

DOI: 10.4324/9781003538226-11

## To Heal Is to Make Whole

To heal comes from an old German word, *healen*, which is the root of interrelated concepts: healthy, holy, whole. To heal a system is to make it whole. To heal a system is more than repairing a broken part or to restoring it to some previous functional status. To heal denotes a profound sense of unification and coherence. To heal healthcare is to reduce its fractures. To heal a social system, which is inspired by human thought and animated by human hands, is a commitment to systemic transformation.

## Healing the Healthcare System

Just as clinical medicine follows a sequence of events for healing, so does systems thinking. Both begin with making the correct diagnosis. It should be obvious by now that piecemeal healthcare reform is the same as the wrong diagnosis in medicine. For healthcare, making the correct diagnosis means recognizing and addressing underlying structural issues and mental models that cause the undesirable events. Because healthcare is a complex system, this means understanding the entire causal chain between undesirable events—inefficiency, ineffectiveness, and inequity—and their root causes.

It's an examination that drills down in step-wise sequence from the undesirable events, to patterns, to structure, and ends with mental models. The diagnostic evaluation also includes making sure the right parts are present, that is, no crucial part is missing, damaged, or obsolete. Lastly, this includes assuring the system's boundaries are the right size. Healthy boundaries include only the essential parts and leave everything else outside. Healthy boundaries are protective—neither too rigid nor too porous.

Because social systems are held together by human relationships, to heal a system is to alter human relationships. To include all Americans means "hitching" together fractured parts into a unified whole. Seemingly easy. However, the reality is more challenging for healing means altering the flow of information and resources among and between the stakeholder groups in order to benefit the whole, not the strongest parts.

Historically, the greatest fears regarding healthcare reform have to do with the effect the distribution of resources will have on *me*. How will universal care be paid for? What benefits will be covered? Who decides? Can I trust them to include me? And, spoken more privately, why should I pay for my neighbor's care when I don't find him worthy? Thus, it goes without saying that building and improving relationships, prior to policy development, is complicated, extensive, political, and fraught.

## Current Reality

In systems thinking, current reality refers to the actual state of a system, right now. The current reality tree (CRT) is an analytic tool that presents a big picture perspective of a system, much like an apple tree depicts its fruit, branches, trunk, and roots. The CRT is fact based and shows the causal sequence from the undesirable events to their root causes. By showing and analyzing the causal sequence of *multiple* undesirable events, the CRT depicts where multiple factors come together, contributing to the undesirable events, thus indicating where to intervene for the best chances of success. Similar to the Iceberg Model, the CRT connects the events to their root causes. The difference is that the CRT shows the causal linkages among and between multiple undesirable events, whereas the Iceberg Model focuses on one undesirable event at a time.

Because social systems are not inert, like a mechanical watch, but are inspired by human thought and animated by human hands, current reality also involves stakeholder groups being truthful about their relationships with other parts of the system. This means each stakeholder group explains its beliefs and assumptions behind its interpretation of the current events, as well as whatever positive or negative effect the events has on it. Open communication is important to collaboration and cooperation, for instance, the current reality of a patient is not the same as that of a CEO of a large pharmaceutical company. This is why stories are as important as numbers and the why entire ensemble of stakeholder groups must be involved in healing the system. Otherwise, it's the cliché of the six blindmen describing the elephant, when in reality none can see the whole.

Without a doubt, healthcare reform is a political endeavor. However, healing solutions can't happen without social linking. This means having multi-sectional representation of stakeholders, who range from community organizations, to professional associations, to businesses, as well as politicians and policy analysts. With multi-sector engagement, shared interested are identified as are competing values and beliefs. This shared decision-making reduces the risk of ending up with contradicting policies and competitive stakeholders; it increases the opportunity for success. In this era short on trust and heavy on disinformation and gaslighting, it's a tall order, indeed, to integrate healthcare's competitive parts into a unified whole. The efficiency, effectiveness, and equity of peer countries' healthcare systems prove that the work is worth the effort, however.

## Current Reality and the Fractured Healthcare System

It's tempting to solve for the undesirable effect de jour, even though sixty years of failed cost containment "solutions" have proven, piecemeals solutions don't work. It's also tempting to ignore the analysis and jump to a solution. Sometimes it's wise to go slow to go fast, which means revisiting healthcare's current reality. The first reality is a healthy system is efficient, effective, equitable, and produces its product. That the U.S. healthcare system violates all four hallmarks of a healthy system are undesirable events.

The second reality is the U.S. healthcare system is honeycombed with fractures. Two important fractures were built into its original design. One was the separation between private medical care for those who could pay and public health for the indigent. The other was the separation of physical health from mental health. Since then, healthcare's structure has been further fractured by the continual additions of new forms of health insurance for special interest groups. Today, there is employer-sponsored insurance for qualified workers, Medicare for seniors, Medicare for dialysis patients, Medicaid for qualified indigent, workers' compensation for qualified job-related injuries, etc. With each add-on came a different slate of covered benefits for patients and reimbursement rules for providers. Today, there are about 1,100 different plans, all of which vary enormously, are ever changing, and further fracture an unstable system.

The third reality in the causal chain of events is the various insurance-related fracture lines are linked to the two structural determinants of health: (1) SOCIOECONOMIC & POLITICAL CONTEXT and (2) SOCIOECONOMIC POSITION. These linkages contribute to healthcare's inefficiency. However, they are also major contributors to healthcare's ineffectiveness and inequities. The first, the SOCIOECONOMIC & POLITICAL CONTEXT, determines the basket of health producing resources within the community (think zip code). The second, SOCIOECONOMIC POSITION, determines who has access to these resources and benefits, and who is excluded and suffers.

Finally, the causal chain of undesirable events shows the root causes of the many fractures. The roots are the mental models, which include deeply held beliefs such as the parts are more important than the whole; healthcare is a consumer product, available to those who can afford it; the definition of health as the ability to work; market segregation and competition can control costs; states' rights; and social Darwinism, to name a few.

Social systems are held together by interlocking networks of human relationship and these relationships determine the flow of information and resources among and between the parts. Therefore, current reality also includes analyzing the flow of information and resources among and between stakeholder groups. For instance, according to the WHO, universal coverage means "all people have access to the full range of quality health services they need, when and where they need them, without financial hardship. Access covers the full continuum of essential health services, from health promotion to prevention, treatment, rehabilitation and palliative care."[1]

But what are essential services and who gets to decide? Similarly, since hearing, vision, dental and mental health are important to overall health, should they be considered essential services? Similarly, at the policy level, what are the optimal spending allocations across the continuum of essential services, by medical specialty, and by geographic region; who gets to decide? Plus, what is the optimal allocation to assure an adequate supply of doctors, nurses, clinicians, and facilities, as well as for research and development? Finally, should all of the money be spent on medical care, or should a portion be devoted to improving the social determinants of health?

## Current Reality and Boundaries

Since the diagnostic evaluation also includes making sure the rights parts are present and the system's boundaries are the right size, it's useful to review the structure of the U.S. healthcare system and its boundaries. The structure of the U.S. healthcare system was organized when infectious diseases and industrial trauma were the leading cause of death. Based on the beliefs and science of the time, the four essential parts of its structure were (1) the healer, a licensed physician, (2) the patient, someone with a biological problem, (3) the disease, biological pathology, and (4) the treatment, pharmaceutical drugs, and surgery. At the time of its formation, healthcare was a cottage industry. Doctors charged what the market would bear, with the wealthier paying more and the poorer paying less, and hospitals were just emerging in curative importance.

Because health insurance was then in the future, it was outside healthcare's boundaries where it remains today. Although outside healthcare's boundaries, the health insurance industry is tightly connected to but separate from the U.S. healthcare system. According to this arrangement, the health insurance industry has much more control over the operation of healthcare system than the system has over the insurance industry.

Other wealthy countries solved this power imbalance power by bringing health insurance inside healthcare's boundaries, vis-à-vis a global budget. By bringing separate elements into a cohesive whole, they unified their healthcare system. By doing so, peer countries gained control over total healthcare costs. Unification also assured the equitable distribution of essential services to all their citizens. Making their universal systems non-profit and integrating health insurance into the whole assure the money goes to sustaining the parts inside the system instead of going to investors and stockholders who are outside the system, or to buy political influence.

## Current Reality and Updating the Cause of Disease

The British epidemiologist Thomas McKeown was the first to show that the types of sickness follow historical periods. Much has changed since the infancy of the U.S. healthcare system. Infectious diseases and trauma have been replaced by chronic diseases as the leading causes of death. Since COVID-19, mental disorders are also on the rise. Just as infectious diseases were once associated with squalor and unsanitary living conditions, chronic diseases are associated with today's living conditions. Whereas infectious diseases were caused by germs rampant in an unsanitary environment, chronic diseases are caused by stress of living in poverty, racism, and unsafe environments, or the two structural social determinants of health (SDOH). Just as germs can lead to biological pathology so does stress. Unhealthy living conditions keep the body's stress response turned on. Long term, unmitigated, low-level stress eventually damages vital organs, including the brain, eventually leading to chronic diseases and mental health disorders.

Relative to other wealthy countries, there's been a notable downward trend in the U.S. for almost every measure of physical and mental health status, since the 1980s. The decline in status is noticeable for men and women, the young and the old, rich and poor, and all races. And, it's attributed to the structural SDOH, especially income inequality, racism, environmental pollution, as well as the disappearance of social policies that once protected low-income Whites.

Although Centers for Medicare and Medicaid (CMS), the governmental payer for about 150 million Americans, has made health equity a strategic goal, the majority of its strategic initiatives involves hospitals and the delivery of care.[2] This tacitly expands healthcare's boundaries to include the two structural SDOH—SOCIOECONOMIC

& POLITICAL CONTEXT and SOCIOECONOMIC POSITION. However, the reality is 80% of the determinants of health fall outside healthcare's control. It's erroneous to believe that hospitals and physicians can treat, and certainly not cure, today's unhealthy living conditions. The reality is unhealthy living condition and economic exclusion from healthcare arise from policies that are outside healthcare's boundaries and outside healthcare's control.

Speaking at the Philadelphia Population Health Colloquium in 2023, Paul Keckley, a health consultant, summarized three things peer countries have in common to achieve better health outcomes at a lower cost than the U.S.[3]

- **The other countries had global budgets for healthcare.** Those countries decided that "there's a fixed amount of money we're going to spend," Keckley said. "You think that's going to happen [here]"?
- **The other countries had national standards of care.** "There was a standard of care that the government oversaw," he said. "We don't [have that] … We let everybody determine what's appropriate care, and then we defend it."
- **The other countries made primary care the central form of care.** However, there was a caveat to that, said Keckley: "It wasn't [about] health *or* social services. It was health *and* social services, funded directly by taxes at 2.5 times what we spend in the U.S. on social services, and in which behavioral and physical medicine, prophylactic dentistry, and over-the-counter and prescription drugs were integrated into those models of primary health. That sounded pretty good to me."

## Human Beings and Their Systems Are Mutually Enfolded

The conceptual, policy, and methodological changes needed to make the U.S. healthcare system more efficient, effective, and equitable are well known. The historical resistance to healthcare reform from those who profit from the current system is also well known. If healthcare were simply a mechanical production line, reform would be as easy as, say, removing an outmoded section, adding some new gears, and lengthening the drive chain.

The reality is quite different. Stakeholders and the healthcare system are mutually enfolded, including the insurance industry which, structurally, operates from outside healthcare's boundaries. Unlike a mechanical production line, healthcare is an organic system, organized by human thought and composed of real people with long memories and strong feelings, who are tightly hitched to their roles, rules, and rewards. They are also hitched to each other in well-established patterns. Resistance arises because of fear of loss and because there's comfort and safety in the familiar, even when the problems are noticeable and uncomfortable.

Ineluctably, to heal the U.S. healthcare system, or to reduce the multiple fractures honeycombing the system, is to adopt a universal healthcare system that is unified by a global budget. A universal healthcare system is more complex than the status quo. Because social systems are held together by human relationships, a universal healthcare system most likely means more complex roles and responsibilities for many of the stakeholder groups. These are big personal changes, for even positive change means new ways of thinking and acting. New tends to come with personal losses, such as the loss of the old, familiar, and comfortable, or worse—the loss of wealth, power, and/or prestige. In a competitive society, few things make us more insecure that the unknown, more anxious than our own awkwardness with the unfamiliar, and more fearful than our vulnerability to loss.

### Objective or Mechanistic Changes

Honeycombed with multiple fractures, the U.S. healthcare system functions like an amalgam of seemingly independent parts, making it easy for stakeholders to be like the six blind men and the elephant. Because the fractures function like blindfolds, stakeholders do not to see the U.S. healthcare system as a whole. Hence, the long stream of historic attempts to "fix the broken part" is understandable. For the past fifty years there's been a steady stream of new and random legislation to control drug costs here, expand Medicaid there, privatize Medicare there, discourage excess utilization with high deductible health plans here, etc.. Blind to the interdependent relationships and unaware of the other groups' roles, rules, and rewards, it makes sense for each stakeholder group to see the other groups as simply another competitive part to be controlled or dominated.

Because stakeholder roles were built into the system a long time ago, stakeholders tend to see the healthcare system as an object separate from themselves, which makes it easy to overlook the tight relationship between human behavior and the system's processes. There's truth to the often-heard excuses, "The computer won't let me." "I'm just following the rules." This oversight conceals the fact that to change either the system or the human behavior is to change them both. Because the interdependency of the relationship is unseen, and therefore, unacknowledged, it's human nature for each stakeholder group to protect their roles and rewards from change. In actuality, however, role behavior cannot change without structural changes to the system, and structural changes, which change the networks of interpersonal relationships, ineluctably alter the stakeholders' roles, rules, and rewards.

### Healing Requires Teamwork

That the U.S. healthcare system is inefficient, ineffective, and inequitable are the classic symptoms of an unhealthy system, a system where the parts neither coordinate nor cooperate well with each other. While it's tempting to blame the stakeholders for their competitive nature and lack of cooperation and coordination, healthcare's dysfunction is inherent in the system's fragmented, for-profit design. Stakeholders, like actors who play Hamlet, are merely playing a role the system assigned to them.

Just as an autoimmune disease, such as lupus, can attack and damage multiple different organs, although some are more vulnerable to damage than others, the data is indisputable that the dysfunction of the U.S. healthcare system is damaging its various stakeholders, albeit in different ways. As we've already seen, about a third of insured patients avoid healthcare because of costs and about 10% of the non-senior public don't have insurance of any kind; too many rural communities lack maternity care; and about 20% of children and teens suffer from mental disorders and mental healthcare is in short supply throughout the U.S.

Physician burnout is endemic in the U.S.; the U.S. doesn't have enough physicians to meet its needs; the physician shortage is especially acute in rural areas; cuts to Medicare reimbursement are forcing some physicians to close their practices to seniors; and about a third of nursing students have no intention of going into bedside nursing. Finally, 40% U.S. hospitals are struggling financially, post-COVID-19, due to ongoing staffing crisis, inflation, and rising pharmaceutical costs. To make matters worse, hospitals' financial struggles are compounded by Medicare and Medicaid reimbursement that is less than the cost of care and by private insurers who have become skillful at denying payment for care. Bottom line, despite healthcare's huge costs–$4.5 trillion—the structure of the U.S. healthcare system is damaging to patients, physicians, and hospitals, alike. The evidence is clear and indisputable.

To heal is to make things whole. To heal the U.S. healthcare system is to integrate the system's fragmented, competitive parts into a cooperative whole. The challenge is for each stakeholder group to change enough so it contributes to the harmony of the whole. To do so requires representatives from all the stakeholders to be at the table. Simply put, the U.S. healthcare system is too large, too complex, and involves too many disparate, competitive stakeholders for one stakeholder group, or even a few groups, to have all the answers or to speak for everyone else. This is especially true when trust is in short supply and when stakeholders, who hold high socioeconomic positions, such as physicians, politicians, and insurance CEOs, are used to using their position to control the agenda and protect themselves from change.

## The Tragedy of the Commons

The parable of the "Tragedy of the Commons" is a story about protecting self-interests. It's also a story about incremental healthcare reform. The parable describes an aggregate of shepherds who graze their sheep on a common pasture. Each shepherd knows that it is in his self-interest to increase the size of his herd, because each additional animal increases his profit, while the damage done to the pasture is shared by everyone. Eventually, the pasture is overgrazed, the sheep don't fatten, the ewes have fewer lambs, and the profits to each shepherd begin to drop. By the time the shepherds realize their problem, it's too late to save the commons.

The moral of the story is that the whole sustains the parts. However, there are other lessons to be drawn. One is, selfishness pays off, at least in the short run. When the pasture runs out of grass, the losers are the shepherds who have been conscientious, who have done their part to maintain the integrity of the whole. In contrast, the winners are those who have grazed the most sheep, ending up with the most profits. They have more resources and can move to new and better pastures, if there are any. The second lesson is, since the commons and the shepherds are mutually enfolded, the whole needs to protect itself. This is done by mutual accountability where, together, the shepherds establish rules to restrict consumption and consequences for overuse. The final lesson is that the tragedy cannot be solved until a critical mass of shepherds adopt a new, holistic, way of thinking and acting to protect the whole. Plus, the rate of adoption must be great enough to maintain this mutually enfolded whole.

## North Star

Once upon a time sailors used the north star for navigation. North stars are reference points and critical for long journeys. Just as the north star helped sailors identify their location, track, and stay their course, healing the healthcare system also requires a north star. North stars are aspirational. In systems thinking, north stars represent a clear and shared purpose. Here, clarity means a shared mental model of the future, that is, one, integrated system that is efficient, effective, and equitable. Clarity also means jointly agreed upon goals that protect the whole, not optimize a part or two. Finally, clarity provides the rationale for healing, that is, to look deeper than the current events and be willing to replace the mental models, which are driving the dysfunctional behavior of the present healthcare system.

North stars are the antidote to the Tragedy of the Commons. North stars are motivational. Representing a clear and shared purpose and jointly agreed goals, north stars motivate stakeholders to learn, adapt, work through setbacks, as well as help each other stay the course during periods of inevitable chaos, confusion, and contretemps.

In the midst of chaos, north stars help stakeholders sort through the confusion of too many choices, and see novel, sustainable opportunities. North stars help stakeholders identify opportunities for optimizing relationships, while shifting the stakeholders' focus away from protecting their personal gain. Because they provide a shared mental model of the future, north stars also help stakeholders move forward in the same direction, despite differences in roles, responsibilities, and rewards. By following the north star, stakeholders track where they are on the healing journey. Tracking reveals either opportunities for sustainable forward movement or for course correction.

## Seeing the Whole

Because the U.S. healthcare system is composed of an aggregate of stakeholders whose relationships affect and are affected by the system, healing the U.S. healthcare system requires bringing a critical mass of all of the stakeholders into the journey. Talking together provides a forum for each stakeholder group to describe its perception of the U.S. healthcare system. In systems thinking, talking together is how each group's mental model of healthcare is made explicit and public. This is important because, like the blind men and the elephant, stakeholders don't share the same mental model. Generally speaking, each group's model arises from its education and socioeconomic status, and the regulations, technology, traditions, education, and experiences common to the group. For instance, physicians' lived experiences and expectations of the healthcare system are different from those of patients, and different yet from the experiences and expectations of the insurance industry.

By surfacing the mental models, stakeholders can see what they hold in common, as well as their differences. The collective insights reveal the root causes of the inequities, inefficiencies, and ineffectiveness of the current system. This more complete and deeper way of seeing shows why previous efforts to reform the U.S. healthcare system have failed, despite reformers' good intentions. Exposing root causes also removes the temptation to impose quick, piecemeal, and/or superficial fixes, or fixes that protect some stakeholder groups at others' expense.

Such insights hold the potential for the future. They help explain what causes some relationships to work, what needs to be improved, what needs to be eliminated, and what new relationships are needed for the system to become more efficient, effective, and equitable. This information helps stakeholders organize and integrate actions to heal systemic fractures. In short, only by seeing the whole can stakeholders clearly understand the root causes of the current dysfunction of the healthcare system and identify potential strategies for healing.

### Healing Is a Public and Private Experience

For the stakeholders, healing the U.S. healthcare system is both a public and private experience. While each stakeholder group brings novel information to the conversation, in actuality the information is brought by human mouths, is heard by human ears, and is animated by human hands. It follows then that healing the U.S. healthcare system is both a public and private experience, governed by a critical mass of stakeholders willing to adopt new ways of thinking and acting in order to protect the whole.

Every significant change is preceded by some force that disrupts the status quo. For patients, a severe illness can be a game changer. Unraveling familiar roles and depending on others for information, the need for help and support threatens the patient's habitual autonomy, as well as how he prefers to perceive himself and the world. These threats leave the patient, at the start of his healing journey, with a terrifying sense of vulnerability. Like recovery from a serious illness, this same sense of vulnerability is inherent to healthcare reform. From a mechanical perspective, for healthcare to be more effective, efficient, and equitable simply means a rewiring of stakeholders' relationships so that relationships are more effective, efficient, and equitable. However, from a human perspective, rewiring stakeholders' relationships means changes to stakeholders' roles, responsibilities, and rewards, which are very, very *personal.*

### Compassion

Compassion means to suffer or experience with—to actually feel another's weal and woe. Compassion is more than pity, sympathy, or mercy; they contain elements of patronization. Compassion connotes a sense of shared humanity, an active regard for everyone's health and well-being, and recognition that relationships are reciprocal. Thus, compassion is the ability to act for the greater good, to contribute to the well-being of the whole, supplanting the temptation to blame, control, withdraw, or take advantage of the sufferer.

Compassion requires emotional maturity, a key ingredient if the stakeholders are to not succumb to the chaos, momentary losses, and distrust of their north star.

Emotional maturity is not a function of the stakeholder's socioeconomic position but is a function of the stakeholder's capacity to tolerate vulnerability, ambiguity, and anomie. Emotionally mature stakeholders have the capacity to model vulnerability by telling their own truth and to accept the emotional and intellectual tension that is experienced when mental models reveal the myriad inconsistent and incongruent perceptions regarding the relationships that form the healthcare system. Because they understand that the external may mirror their own inner world, emotionally mature stakeholders are able to stay calm, courageous, and compassionate. Bluntly speaking, emotionally mature stakeholders don't suffer burnout or compassion fatigue.

Emotionally mature stakeholders understand that new information often feels like betrayal, that humans are emotional before they are rational. Emotionally mature stakeholders wish to relieve suffering, instead of defending the status quo or blaming others. Instead of distrust, there is mutual respect. Instead of seeking self-protection, there's shared purpose and concern for one another's welfare. They have the courage to bridge and link with those "not of their tribe," despite asymmetrical power differences. Instead of needing to control, emotionally mature stakeholders are curious, caring, and willing to experiment. Emotionally mature stakeholders are good at amplifying others' strengths and organizing opportunities for change. They are able to stay focused on the north star instead of the chaos. Instead of withdrawing, they have the capacity to learn from failures and remain engaged even when nothing seems to hold. Emotionally mature stakeholders are good at reinforcing the purpose and aligning roles, goals, metrics, and incentives to support all of the stakeholders and reinforce the purpose of healing a fractured healthcare system.

## Self-Protection and Instability

Systems thinking posits that an unstable system is not able to return to its original state after being perturbed. Instead, as each part attempts to protect itself, the perturbations are amplified, making things worse. Thus, an unstable system is difficult to control and its future actions are less predictable than when it was stable.

Health insurance is supposed to be protective against healthcare's soaring costs. The reality is even people with health insurance worry about costs. Insurance doesn't protect them from catastrophic medical expenses, such as paying for their 20% of a million-dollar bill or paying for the first $10,000 of their high deductible plan. Americans are finding healthcare's soaring costs untenable. According to the fourth quarter Keckley poll, "69% of those polled believe the U.S. healthcare system is fundamentally flawed and in need of major change; 60% believe it puts profits over patients; 74% believe price controls are needed; and 76% think politicians avoid dealing with healthcare issues because they're complex and politically risky."[4]

While the poll supports the desire for a healthcare system that is effective, efficient, and equitable, and there are periodic calls to "repeal and replace Obamacare," what is lacking, so far, is any kind of cooperative effort for a universal healthcare system. Although grassroots efforts in twenty states are working for Medicare for

All for their specific state, which is, simply speaking, how the Canadian system began, with one province leading the way, it looks like the powerful stakeholders are already engaged in self-protection. For instance, at the October, 2023, Interim Meeting of the American Medical Association (AMA), participants agreed that the current system is broken, but were divided as to whether a single-payer system would either crater the system or increase access. AMA members also blamed Medicare for not keeping up with inflation and threatened not to treat Medicare patients. Some drug companies and the U.S. Chamber of Commerce are suing the federal government over the new Medicare price negotiations that is limited to *ten* drugs. And, in the summer of 2023, the American Hospital Association (AHA), through a *Wall Street Journal* editorial, asked Congress to halt cuts to Medicare reimbursement, extend healthcare coverage subsidies, and hold insurance companies accountable for improper business practices. Two of the largest insurance companies, Cigna and Humana, are talking about merging, which would reduce competition to hospitals and could raise costs and reduce choices for the public. Hospitals continue to merge, with fifteen large hospital systems now controlling about a third of the market. Health insurers and private equity continue to employ physicians, with United Health Group now employing 10% of all US physicians.

Also, there are several other, broader proposals for "fixing" the healthcare system. November, 2023, Representative Ro Khanna (D-CA) introduced the State-Based Universal Health Care Act. The proposed legislation creates a waiver that allows states to bundle all their healthcare spending to fund a state-level single-payer system. In their book, *We've Got You Covered: Rebooting American Health Care*, Einav and Finkelstein propose "universal coverage for a basic set of medical services [that is free at the point of care] and the option to buy additional, supplemental coverage in a well-designed market,"[5] which creates a two-tiered medical system. Some prominent Republican congressmen have recommended significant cuts to Medicare. And, as part of his re-election campaign, former President Trump has said that, he's looking at alternatives to the Affordable Care Act.

The current reality is sobering. To date, the evidence shows a stronger picture of self-protection than protecting the whole. To date, there's no evidence of a national coalition representing *all* stakeholder groups nor is there evidence of a north star to guide stakeholders toward a more efficient, effective, equitable healthcare system—for everyone. Unfortunately, the evidence indicates another round of piecemeal solutions, promising the likelihood that the Tragedy of the Commons will be repeated, again, adding more fractures to an already unstable system.

## Hope

According to the Greek myth of Pandora's Box, there is always hope. The myth speaks to the paradox of healthcare reform. The story is about Pandora who was given a box that was not hers to open. Similar to the phrase, "opening a can of worms," Pandora, in her naïve curiosity, opened the box and all kinds of awful problems flew out to bedevil the world. According to the myth, Hope, by remaining in the box, is a paradoxical creature. According to one interpretation, Hope is simply another bedevilment that didn't have time to fly away before Pandora closed the lid. Another interpretation claims Hope is a virtue, but its imprisonment symbolizes that life is bleak, difficult, and without hope. Others say Hope remained in the box because its presence is an energizing virtue, a winged creature, bright and full of light. Its brightness symbolizes light—a north star lighting the way when the current reality is bleak and dark. And, its wings symbolize action in the pursuit of personal or collective healing.

Hope is not magical thinking, or toxic positivity. Hope is a beacon in the darkness. Hope symbolizes the ability to envision a healthier future, see potential in the darkness, and trust the right actions will lead to positive outcomes. Hope is not unrealistic expectations. Hope is the realistic understanding that healthy children are our future and healthy people are vital to national security and a robust economy. Hope is the understanding that I and my neighbor are more alike than different. Needing access to healthcare is one of our basic similarities. Hope symbolizes the motivation to persevere even when the expected outcome is not guaranteed. Hope is a positive emotion that broadens our thinking, fosters creativity and courage, and strengthens social connections. Hope is healing.

## Questions for the Reader

The questions provide an opportunity to examine your own mental models and values and to imagine other stakeholders' beliefs, fears, and values.

1 Knowing that some form of universal healthcare redresses healthcare's efficiency, effectiveness, and equity problems and knowing the greatest barrier to change are fears about the effect the redistribution of resources will have on *me.* What are your greatest fears regarding a universal healthcare system: cost to me, fewer covered benefits, loss of choice, others may get something they haven't earned; other? Why do you believe this; what might other stakeholder groups fear.
2 Assuming universal healthcare is adopted, which major stakeholder groups of the existing system—patients, doctors, hospitals, insurers, and pharmaceutical companies—might lose the most? Which might benefit the most? Why; what might others think.
3 Without a doubt, healthcare reform is a political endeavor and multi-sector engagement is vital for reform to succeed. What stakeholder groups do you believe should be at the table: representatives from healthcare's professional associations, big business, religious and social service organization, politicians, policy analysts, the public, others? Who do you trust to speak for you? Why; what might others believe?
4 To heal the U.S. healthcare system is to integrate the system's fragmented, competitive parts into a cooperative whole. The challenge is for each stakeholder group to change enough so it contributes to the harmony of the whole. What are the challenges to change your stakeholder group might face; what challenges might other groups face? Why; what might others believe?
5 To what extent are you responsible for the well-being of others? To what extent does society have an obligation to meet your needs? Why; what might others believe?

6 Knowing that sooner or later everyone needs healthcare; that my health affects my coworkers' health; that healthy people are the backbone of national security and the sinew of a strong economy, is this knowledge enough for polarized groups to find common ground? If yes, why? If not, where is common ground to be found?
7 Who might you bond, bridge, and/or link with to facilitate bringing some form of universal healthcare to all Americans? How would you do this?
8 How do we become more compassionate, knowing that there are limits to what we can do for others and that they can do for us, yet knowing that we need each other?
9 A north star brings new perspectives, knowledge, beliefs, and actions, which are accompanied by loss or fear of loss, on the part of stakeholders. What losses might you fear? What losses might other stakeholders fear? Would the guarantee of a more efficient, effective, equitable healthcare system mitigate these fears? Why; what might others believe?

## Notes

1 Universal Health Coverage. www.who.int/health-topics/univer.
2 CMS Strategic Plan Health Equity Fact Sheet. https://www.cms.gov/files/document/health-equity-factsheet-2023.pdf.
3 Want better health outcomes? Check out what other countries do. (2023, September 19). *MedPage Today*. https://www.medpagetoday.com/meetingcoverage/phc/106393.
4 Keckley Poll: The public is fed up with the health care system…so what else is new. (2023, November 20). *The Keckley Report*. https://www.paulkeckley.com/the-keckley-report.
5 Einav, L., & Finkelstien, A. (2023) *We've Got You Covered: Rebooting American Health Care*. New York: Portfolio/Penguin. p. xx.

# Acknowledgments

Why healthy relationships are important is one of the themes of this book. People with strong social connections are healthier and live longer. They are also happier. The stability and performance of social systems, like healthcare, depend on the goodness of the relationships holding the system together. Therefore, it's a pleasure to thank Sue Arambel, Joyce Corcoran, Carol Farina, Catherine Ito, Ken Kaufman, Leesa Kuhlman, Carolyn Molson, Bernadette Prinster, Nancy Stauffer, and Joanna Tardoni. You read for me and sent me many of the examples about healthcare's failures. Although the market is replete with books about what's wrong with the U.S. healthcare system and what can be done to fix the issue *de jour*, it was encouraging to hear you say, "I wish I'd known that," "Why isn't this ever mentioned in the popular media"? and "Keep writing."

By exploring healthcare as a whole system, the book shows that cost, quality, access, and health disparities are inter-related and cannot be solved by attempting to optimize whatever is the issue of the day. Obviously, I believe the solution is some form of a non-profit, universal healthcare system. It's a fraught and unlikely solution, to be sure. Although this book doesn't represent their thinking, conversation with Josh Hanes, Vice President of the Wyoming Hospital Association; Sue Ellen Wagner, Vice President of Trustee Engagement, AHA; and Banu Symington, M.D. were instrumental in clarifying my own.

A special thanks to the members of the Board of Trustees of Memorial Hospital of Sweetwater County (MHSC), especially Marty Kelsey, Richard Mathey, and Kandi Pendleton who read various sections of the book. Ed Tardoni, another board member, deserves special thanks for reading the book in its entirety, challenging some of my assumptions, and having faith in me. I also want to thank the hospital staff. Healthcare is not just a business; it is a calling. Your care and compassion—the defining quality of the patient-care giver relationship—help alleviate suffering and improve health outcomes. I am inspired by your dedication and am proud to be part of the hospital.

Those of us who write non-fiction books depend upon the experiences, data, and assumptions of others, not just our own. The prevalence of articles about healthcare's cost, quality, access, and health disparities problems indicates the U.S. healthcare system doesn't work well for the vast majority of its stakeholders. Some of my daily readings came from Medpage Today, the various Becker Reviews, and

JAMA online publications. Also read regularly were The Keckley Report, Kaufman Hall reports, and Doximity. Thus, a deep bow of appreciation to their editors and reporters.

This book wouldn't have happened without the support of Routledge Publishing. They saw the value of looking at healthcare's problems and the solution through the lens of systems thinking. I am grateful to them for making this book possible and to the staff who made it better.

Even with the help of those mentioned, this book couldn't have been written without the love and support of my husband, Robert Sowada. Finally, any mistakes are solely mine.

# Index

Note: *Italicized* pages refer to figures.

For Product Safety Concerns and Information please contact our EU representative GPSR@taylorandfrancis.com Taylor & Francis Verlag GmbH, Kaufingerstraße 24, 80331 München, Germany

**Batch number: 10397794**

Printed by Printforce, the Netherlands